Mental Health and Social Policy in Ireland

Social policy in Ireland
Other titles published by UCD Press:

Contemporary Irish Social Policy
edited by SUZANNE QUIN, PATRICIA KENNEDY,
ANNE MATTHEWS, and GABRIEL KIELY

Irish Social Policy in Context
edited by GABRIEL KIELY, ANNE O'DONNELL,
PATRICIA KENNEDY and SUZANNE QUIN

Disability and Social Policy in Ireland
edited by SUZANNE QUIN and BAIRBRE REDMOND

Theorising Irish Social Policy
edited by BRYAN FANNING, PATRICIA KENNEDY
GABRIEL KIELY and SUZANNE QUIN

Irish Social Policy in Focus
edited by BRYAN FANNING and MICHAEL RUSH
(forthcoming)

COMHAIRLE CHONTAE ÁTHA CLIATH THEAS
SOUTH DUBLIN COUNTY LIBRARIES

STEWARTS HOSPITAL BRANCH
TO RENEW ANY ITEM TEL:

Items should be returned on or before the last date below. Fines,
as displayed in the Library, will be charged on overdue items.

First published 2005
by University College Dublin Press
Newman House
86 St Stephen's Green
Dublin 2
Ireland
www.ucdpress.ie

ISBN 1-904558-32-1

Cataloguing in Publication data
available from the British Library

Typeset in Ireland in
Adobe Garamond and Trade Gothic
by Elaine Burberry, Bantry, Co. Cork
Text design by Lyn Davies
Index by Jane Rogers
Printed in England on acid-free
paper by Antony Rowe Ltd

Contents

Health Boards

Important note
The administration of the health services was taken
over by the Health Service Executive in January 2005
and the term 'health board' is no longer in use.

Contributors to this volume

MARY ALLEN is currently Director of the Postgraduate Social Work Programme in University College Dublin. She has worked in community work and community activism in Africa and Brazil, as a senior medical social worker in St James's Hospital Dublin and as manager of the training unit of Women's Aid. Her research interests include suicide and non-fatal suicidal behaviour, and violence against women in intimate relationships.

MICHAEL BERGIN is a lecturer in nursing at the Department of Nursing, Waterford Institute of Technology. He previously worked as a psychiatric nurse in the Kilkenny Mental Health Services for over twenty years, having held positions of clinical nurse manager, community mental health nurse and project officer for the integration of the Carlow/Kilkeny Mental Health Services. His current research interests are in community mental health and enduring and persistent mental health problems and gender.

JEAN CLARKE is a senior lecturer in the Department of Nursing, Dublin City University. Her research interests include nursing care with special emphasis on oppression and caring, and paediatric palliative care. She is a former public health nurse and has worked in nursing education since 1987. She is a member of Sigma Theta Thau and a former member of the editorial board of the *Journal of Community Nursing*. She has published in the areas of public health nursing and the gendered role of nursing within health-care organisations.

PAULINE CONROY is a social policy analyst and director of the research and design company, Ralaheen Ltd. She has lectured in European Social Policy in University College Dublin for many years. Dr Conroy has conducted research into the costs of disability in Ireland, on the recruitment of people with disabilities into the Irish public service and has worked with the International Labour Office on a code of practice for the employment of people with disabilities.

MARY DRURY, as a medical social worker at St James's Hospital, was attached to the Memory Clinic at the Mercer Institute for Research on Ageing and worked closely with patients who had been diagnosed with a dementia and their families. She was interim director of the newly established Dementia Services Information and Development Centre in 1998 and became the Centre's first education officer until 2003 when she returned to the Social Work Department in St James's Hospital as Deputy Manager. She is currently senior social worker in Leopardstown Park Hospital.

IRIS ELLIOTT has worked as a social worker in therapeutic, community development and statutory mental health services in England and Ireland. She has also worked as a health promotion specialist with post-primary schools in Dublin, Wicklow and Kildare. Following two years with the Institute of Public Health in Ireland developing trans-national and national health policy, she now works in the National Disability Authority, Ireland as a senior policy and public affairs advisor.

VIVIAN GEIRAN joined the Probation and Welfare Service in 1987 and served as a probation officer on a number of prison and community-based teams. He was also senior probation and welfare officer in the Research and Statistics Unit and Drug Court team. Since becoming an assistant principal probation and welfare officer in 2002, he has headed the Homeless Offenders Strategy Team (HOST). He also lectures on the Masters in Social Work programme in Trinity College, Dublin, is co-editor of the *Irish Probation Journal* and is a member of the editorial committee of the *Irish Social Worker* journal.

NICK GOULD is Professor of Social Work at the University of Bath, UK. He is a registered social worker and maintains an involvement in mental health practice. In addition to mental health, he researches and publishes in the fields of professional learning, evidence-based practice, and the impacts of new technology in human services.

ELIZABETH HICKEY is self-employed as a psychotherapist and social researcher. She is an occasional lecturer in the Department of Social Policy and Social Work in University College Dublin and in the Department of Applied Social Studies in NUI Maynooth. She is also a practice tutor in the Department of Social Policy and Social Work, UCD. She was previously employed as a probation and welfare officer by the Department of Justice, Equality and Law Reform and as head medical social worker by the then North Eastern Health Board. She has published on a diverse range of subjects including the criminal justice system and women's health. She has a particular interest in women's mental health.

PATRICIA KENNEDY is a senior lecturer in the Department of Social Policy and Social Work. She is co-founder of the Irish Social Policy Association. She is particularly interested in social policy from a feminist perspective and has taught and written widely on the subject. Her most recent publications include *Maternity in Ireland: A Woman-Centred Perspective* (Liffey, 2002) and *Motherhood in Ireland: Creation and Context* (Mercier, 2003).

JOE MORAN worked with refugees and asylum seekers in the public and voluntary sector for almost ten years. He currently teaches social policy at the Waterford

Institute of Technology and at the Institute of Technology, Carlow – Wexford Campus. He studied at University College Cork, Trinity College Dublin, University of Liverpool and the Institute of Public Administration.

SUZANNE QUIN is a senior lecturer in the Department of Social Policy and Social Work and Director of the PhD in Social Work Structured Programme at University College Dublin. She has worked in St Vincent's Hospital, the Eastern Health Board and as Head of the Social Work Department in the National Rehabilitation Hospital. She has also lectured in social policy in Trinity College Dublin and in the Institute of Public Administration. She has co-edited a number of books for UCD Press including the companion volume *Disability and Social Policy in Ireland* (2003).

BAIRBRE REDMOND is a senior lecturer in the Department of Social Policy and Social Work and Associate Dean of Teaching and Learning, Faculty of Human Sciences at University College Dublin. Her research and teaching interests include disability issues and the development of innovative teaching techniques for health and social service professionals. She is Chair of the Complaints Committee of the Advertising Standards Authority of Ireland and she is also a member of the Private Residential Tenancies Board of Ireland.

VALERIE RICHARDSON is a senior lecturer in the Department of Social Policy and Social Work, University College Dublin. She is the Irish expert on the European Observatory on the Social Situation, Demography and the Family. A graduate of the University of Wales, she undertook her postgraduate professional training in social work in the University of Edinburgh.

VICTORIA RICHARDSON is a qualified social worker currently employed as the psychiatric social worker in St Vincent's University Hospital, Dublin. She has practised in the field of child protection and child guidance and has undertaken research on the service needs of mothers caring for children with profound disabilities.

MIKE TIMMS is Academic Director in the Centre for Disability Studies at University College Dublin. He has worked as senior clinical psychologist in the Eastern Health Board, the National Rehabilitation Board (NRB) and the National Disability Authority (NDA). In the 1990s, he spent time seconded to various Eastern European countries (Czech Republic, Poland and Slovakia), delivering EU-funded training under the PHARE programme. Earlier in his career, he was highly involved in the move of mental health services to the community, leading a number of outreach initiatives and being involved in the management of community-based hostels for people with mental health difficulties.

Abbreviations

ADHD	Attention Deficit Disorder
ASD	Autistic Spectrum Disorder
CHPS	Centre for Health Promotion Studies (NUI Galway)
CMH	Central Mental Hospital
CSM	Community sanctions and measures
CSO	Central Statistics Office
DFID	Department for International Development
DSM	Diagnostic and Statistical Manual of Mental Disorders
EC	European Commission
ESRI	Economic and Social Research Institute
ETAS	European Trans-national Alzheimer's Study
HEBS	Health Education Board for Scotland
HIA	Health Impact Assessment
HPU	Health Promotion Unit
HRB	Health Research Board
ICP	Irish College of Psychiatrists
ICD	International Classification of Diseases
ILO	International Labour Office
IMHPA	Implementing Mental Health Promotion Action
IPA	Institute of Public Administration
IPS	Irish Prison Service
LRC	Law Reform Commission
NDA	National Disability Authority
NESC	National Economic and Social Council
NESF	National Economic and Social Forum
NHS	National Health Service (UK)
NSRF	National Suicide Research Foundation
NUIG	National University of Ireland, Galway
NWCI	National Women's Council of Ireland
ODEI	Office of Director of Equality Investigations
OOPEC	Office for Official Publications of the European Communities
PAS	Post Abortion Syndrome
PMDD	Pre-menstrual Dysphoric Disorder
PMS	Pre-menstrual Tension Syndrome
PND	Post Natal Depression
PNDAI	Post Natal Depression Association of Ireland
PSI	Psychological Society of Ireland
PTSD	Post Traumatic Stress Disorder

QNHS	Quarterly National Household Survey
QoL	Quality of Life
QOLA	Quality of Life Analysis
SPIRASI	Asylum Services Initiative
STAKES	National Research and Development Centre, Finland
TCD	Trinity College, Dublin
UCD	University College Dublin
UN	United Nations
UPIAS	Union of Physically Impaired Against Segregation
WHO	World Health Authority

Introduction

Suzanne Quin
Bairbre Redmond

The purpose of this book is to provide a text covering major areas of social policy in relation to mental health in Ireland. The book is aimed at a number of different groups who have a shared interest in mental health and social policy. It will be of interest to students of social policy, including comparative social policy, as well as being relevant to a range of professional training courses for social workers, nurses, doctors and psychologists. The same professional groups engaged in practice with those with mental health problems and their families will find it pertinent. It also has relevance for all agencies engaged in policy creation and implementation in this field including those in the voluntary sector. It will be of interest to service users and their families as consumers, evaluators and critics of what is and what should be provided in the area of mental health in Ireland.

This volume serves as a companion to *Disability and Social Policy in Ireland* published in 2003. Having a separate volume for mental health was considered to be appropriate because mental illness cannot be subsumed under the broad umbrella of disability. Some mental illnesses are acute in their nature and treatment while others fit the definition of disability in that they are chronic conditions that have ongoing psychosocial, economic and practical consequences for those affected and for their families. The very scale of mental illness globally and in the Irish context makes it a suitable topic for a volume in its own right.

Estimates of the prevalence of mental health problems show them to be of significant import globally. According to the World Health Organisation (WHO, 2001a), mental and behavioural disorders are both common (affecting between 20 and 25 per cent of all people at some time in their life) and universal. In relation to Europe, The World Health Organisation estimates that at least five per cent of the population suffers from serious diagnosable mental illnesses and that between 15 and 20 per cent of European adults are affected by more general mental health problems. The association with socio-economic variables is evident, with indications that common mental disorders 'are about

twice as frequent in the lowest income groups compared to the highest'
(European Commission, 2003: 97).

Given the scale and pervasiveness of mental health issues, the question
arises about the level of response in terms of service provision for those affected.
That services are inadequately provided internationally is evidenced by the
World Health Report (WHO, 2001a) which estimated that 'even in countries
with well-established services, fewer than half of those individuals needing care
make use of such services' (2001a: 6). This it attributes to the stigma attached
to mental health problems as well as to the inappropriateness of what was
provided. Even taking this inadequate provision into account, the costs of
providing care for those who do seek treatment are substantial. Studies of
primary care usage indicate that up to 30 per cent of general practitioner
consultations are for mental health problems (European Commission, 2003:
99). Overall, in Europe it is estimated that 'the direct consequences of mental
illness can account for between a third and a half of total health care costs'
(European Commission, 2003: 97).

Apart from the scale and cost of mental health problems, the publication of
this book is timely in that this is an era of significant change in mental health
policy and practice. The National Health Strategy (Department of Health and
Children, 2001b) includes a commitment to developing a policy framework to
update that set out by the policy document *The Psychiatric Services: Planning for
the Future* (Department of Health, 1984). To this end, an Expert Group on
Mental Health Policy was set up in 2003 with a brief to consult all relevant
stakeholders in the creation of a new framework for mental health policy for the
new century. The brief is wide, incorporating models of care, treatment modal-
ities, rehabilitation and the special needs of a range of vulnerable groups. Its
terms of reference are to prepare a comprehensive 10-year policy framework, to
recommend how services should be organised and delivered and the estimated
costs of implementing their proposals. The final report of this Group is due
sometime in 2005 (Department of Health and Children, 2004a).

For too long there had been a reliance on outdated legislation under the
Mental Health Act 1945, but the 1990s became a time of policy development.
The Green Paper in 1992, followed by the White Paper 1995 paved the way for
the introduction of a new Mental Health Act in 2001. This Act was primarily
concerned with creating new processes and safeguards for those who become
involuntary users of mental treatment facilities. The Act also allowed for the
creation of a Mental Health Commission and the replacement of the Inspector
of Mental Hospitals with an inspectorate to take responsibility for overseeing
the standards and practices of mental health services.

It has been in the early years of this century, that the changes planned have
begun to reach fruition. The Mental Health Commission, an independent
statutory body provided for under the Mental Health Act 2001, was established

in 2003. Its brief was to 'promote and foster high standards and good practices in the delivery of mental health services and to ensure that the interests of detained persons are protected' (Department of Health and Children, press release, 14 Mar. 2002). Included in its brief were the office of the Inspector of Mental Health Services and the creation of Mental Health Tribunals (from 2005). The year 2003 also saw the publication of a report by Amnesty International that was critical of policies and services currently provided for those with mental health problems. It argued that the new Mental Health Act 2001 did not go sufficiently far to protect the rights of those involuntarily admitted to in-patient facilities in comparison with similar legislation internationally. Furthermore, it was very critical of both the resourcing and the facilities for the prevention and treatment of mental health in Ireland.

The fact that mental health services are under-resourced, in relation to both size and need, was acknowledged by Brian Lenihan, Minister of State at the Department of Health and Children. In the debate on the Estimates for government spending in 2005 he commented that the additional funding allocated 'shows that this Government is serious about improving the lives of those with a disability or mental health problem . . . I have said on numerous occasions that mental health and disability services need to be improved' (Department of Health and Children, press release, 18 Nov. 2004). That this statement is a truism is well illustrated by the fact that the Primary Care Strategy (Department of Health and Children, 2001e) alluded to lack of resources and personnel to adequately address mental health problems in the community. Inadequate resources has also featured prominently in more recent reports such as that by Amnesty International (2003) and the report of the Irish College of Psychiatrists (2004a) specifically in relation to child and adolescent psychiatry which identifies average waiting time for such services to be a year or more.

Cost was an important factor in the move from institutionally based to community-based settings for the treatment of mental illness which began in the 1960s. Escalating costs, the growing focus on the negative effects of institutionalisation investigated by writers such as Goffman (1961), Townsend (1962), Robb (1967) and the development of psychotropic drugs were together responsible for the large-scale shift to community-based care which began at this time and has continued to the present. This move and its consequences are discussed in a number of chapters in this book. Gould (chapter 1) argues that the institutional/community dichotomy is more complex than is immediately evident. He highlights the critical role of primary care in services for those with mental health problems. Bergin and Clarke (chapter 2) emphasise that the move from institutional care to community care must be accompanied by a move away from a biomedical model of mental health to a bio psychosocial or holistic model of understanding. These authors also highlight the need for re-education and training mental health professionals to develop and maintain effective community care services. Redmond (chapter 12) also notes that the inadequate and inflexible community care services have consistently failed to meet the needs of those with mental health difficulties who are vulnerable to homelessness. As is evident from the chapters' contents, in spite of the focus on community-based services, resources are thinly divided in relation to need.

Another related and more recent trend in mental health policy, in common with health policy overall, is the increasing focus on the importance of health promotion. That mental health promotion is the Cinderella of an under-resourced aspect of health care is evident in Elliott's chapter (chapter 4). This is in spite of the fact that mental health issues affect a sizeable proportion of the population and that the focus is now generally on facilitating good health (including good mental health) to minimise the personal, social and economic costs of curing illness if possible when it occurs. Prevention includes and moves beyond the boundaries of health care into the related fields of social security, employment policy, education policy and housing. Conroy's chapter on mental health and employment (chapter 3) shows the effects of attitudes towards mental illness on employment opportunities for those affected. She illustrates the importance of employment for social and economic integration and examines the effectiveness of legislation in the field of employment in combating issues of stigma in the workplace.

While it is evident from the statistics in the World Health Report (2001a) that mental health is an aspect of health care which impacts on a large section of the overall population, it is also evident that the burden of ill health, as is the case more generally also, falls disproportionately on certain sections of the population. Socio-economic factors, demographic change and lifestyle patterns are all pertinent to understanding the very particular challenges facing vulnerable groups in society. These issues are explored in some depth by a number of authors in this book. For example, Gould (chapter 1) discusses the link between mental illness and poverty, Kennedy and Hickey (chapter 8) in regard to women and Moran (chapter 13) concerning the mental health of Ireland's new communities. Moran discusses the negative impact of low income, poor housing and unemployment on the mental health of immigrants. He also highlights the psychological trauma of the immigration process itself and the distress associated with the social isolation, racism and lack of cultural understanding experienced by these new communities. Redmond (chapter 12) emphasises that lack of affordable housing for young families and the inade-quate after-care plans for young people leaving institutional and foster care result in many vulnerable individuals having to resort to temporary hostel accommodation or to sleeping rough. Such living conditions frequently contribute to depression and to a worsening of any pre-existing mental health problems. They also precipitate or worsen drug and alcohol dependence and involvement with petty crime.

The life cycle aspect of mental illness is another important dimension to be addressed in this volume. Richardson's chapter on children (chapter 5) begins this life course perspective. She highlights the categories of children recognised as being at increased risk of mental illness including urban children living in situation of deprivation, poverty and family breakdown. Also at risk of mental illness are children who have experienced physical or sexual abuse and children with chronic illnesses. Children and young people with intellectual disability may also have an increased risk of developing mental health difficulties and Timms (chapter 10) focuses on the often-neglected needs of those with both intellectual disability and mental illness. Adolescence marks a period of vital developmental importance. Quin and Richardson (chapter 6) look at the specific mental health needs of this group, noting that mental health problems experienced by adolescents have been found to be a good predictor of further problems in adulthood. Drury (chapter 9) examines mental health in old age, noting the need to emphasise sound mental health as one of the main components in 'active ageing'. She also notes that strong links exist between psychological well-being and the prevention of illness in the later stages of the life cycle.

Gender differences in mental health have also been explored in the book. Kennedy and Hickey (chapter 8) examine the particular challenges facing women that render them vulnerable to mental health problems in the context of their socio-economic conditions. Allen (chapter 7) looks at issue of suicide, describing it as both a personal tragedy and a social challenge. She draws attention to the growing incidence of suicide in Ireland, now between eight and nine times what it was in 1970 and the consistent link between mental illness, particularly depression, and suicide. Allen also explores the high level of fatal suicidal behaviour amongst young Irish men, querying its connection with a loss of masculine identity which also expresses itself in serious risk-taking behaviour in the young male population such as heavy drinking, street violence and car crashes. Quin and Richardson (chapter 6) consider the predominantly female mental health issue of eating disorders, noting that eating disorders represent a growing health problem with serious consequences for those affected, both as an immediate risk to life and to long-term health issues. They emphasise the importance of preventative and curative interventions for those with eating disorders as part of a balanced mental health service.

Finally, a number of contributors focus on the complex needs of those with what are termed 'dual diagnoses'– situations where mental health difficulties constitute only part of a multifaceted set of problems. In Timms's chapter (chapter 10) he looks at pertinent issues for individuals with both intellectual disability and mental illness, observing that such individuals may be poorly served by both the services for those with mental illness and the services for the intellectually disabled. Timms recommends both advocacy and person-centred planning to help such individuals express their wishes in terms of life choices and treatment needs. Just as the intellectually disabled population with metal health needs may be inappropriately placed, so also are many of those with mental illness in the prison population. In his chapter 11, Geiran looks at the need to differentiate between treatment and punishment for those with mental illness who offend against the criminal justice system. Geiran also highlights the need to prevent mentally ill individuals becoming habitual offenders and the appropriateness of offering behaviour programmes both in community and custodial settings to mentally ill offenders, many of whom may also have drug or drink related problems.

Poor mental health is no respecter of age, gender or social status and many individuals and their families suffer distress and anguish dealing with mental illness and its consequences. However, this book serves to emphasise how the needs of certain individuals and groups with mental illness have, by virtue of ineffectual or nonexistent policies, been sidelined or ignored for too long. As World Health Ministers stated in 2001, 'mental health care has simply not received until now the level of visibility, commitment and resources of the mental health burden' (WHO, 2001b). The contributors to this book each, in their own way, bring new perspectives not only on the needs of diverse people with mental health needs. Collectively they have also focused on ways in which Irish mental health policies can help develop services and supports which are humane, responsive and equitable.

Chapter 1

International trends in mental health policy

Nick Gould

Introduction

It is increasingly recognised that mental ill-health is a major factor in the global experience of ill-health and disability (Desjarlais et al., 1996). Measuring the so-called Global Burden of Disease with the methodological device of Daily-Adjusted Life Years, the World Health Organisation (WHO, 2002b) has demonstrated the magnitude of the issues:

- Neuropsychiatric disorders comprise 13 per cent of the global burden of disease in 2001.
- Neuropsychiatric disorders contribute 4 of the 10 leading causes of disability.
- Neuropsychiatric disorders contribute 28 per cent of years of life lived with a disability.
- Depression accounts for over 12 per cent of years of life lived with a disability.

If politicians and policy makers are still not persuaded by the magnitude of these prevalence figures, the economic arguments are likely to focus their minds. A study for the European Union calculated that the total costs of mental disorders are about 3–4 per cent of Gross National Product (STAKES, 1999a). The indirect costs of the lack of productivity resulting from exclusion from the labour market multiply even this figure. A study in the UK estimated that the annual cost of mental distress to the national economy was around £77 billion (Sainsbury Centre for Mental Health, 2003a). Without committing us to a narrowly Utilitarian view of this, these figures do provide some kind of proxy of the amount of disruption and distress that are caused in the lives of individuals.

For those of us who are social scientists in the mental health field and of a certain age, these are interesting times. We may well have developed our interest in mental health when anti-psychiatry was in the ascendancy, a broad umbrella for a range of intellectual influences including social constructionism and labelling theory, the Palo Alto school of systems theory and not least R. D. Laing's beguiling cocktail of existentialism, psychedelia and (briefly) Marxist dialectic. For a period in the late 1960s (and remembering of course that the 'Sixties' really happened in the 1970s) it seemed that these influences would synthesise into an irresistible defeat of the hegemony of institutionally based approaches to understanding and treating mental distress. In fact, apart from some exceptions such as Psichiatria Democratica in Italy (a radical alliance of political activists and psychiatrists whose agitation led in 1978 to legislation to close all Italian public mental hospitals) (Donnelly, 1992), this was no more triumphant than the student and worker protests of the same period were in overthrowing the capitalist order. As various commentators have pointed out, anti-psychiatry was more potent as a rallying point for cultural disaffection than it was as a serious response to the complexity and reality of the lives of people who were mentally distressed (Sedgwick, 1982; Miller and Rose, 1986). And some would say that it was ever thus, arguing that the de-institutionalisation of people from large-scale mental institutions across the Western word was instigated by a fiscal crisis of the welfare state (Scull, 1977).

This chapter seeks not to reopen these debates about the reasons for the demise of the asylums but instead reviews the current emergence of new social models in mental health policy, and not least their points of departure from the anti-psychiatry movement of thirty or forty years ago. In the first instance we shall review the broad shifts which have taken place in developed countries concerning mental health policy and institutional arrangements for the delivery of services and, drawing on analyses from neo-institutionalist perspectives in political science, suggest that the emerging picture is more complex and diversified than some of the prophets of convergence would have predicted (Donnelly, 1992; Goodwin, 1997)

The apparent convergence on 'community care' disguises a more subtle mix of processes including separation of treatment and care services, diversification of services to deal with a newly defined and expanded range of mental health problems, and preoccupation with mental disorder as a threat to social order and stability. Within Europe, rather than simple convergence, there is a loose clustering of 'ideal types' of mental health services, partially corresponding to welfare regimes, but individual countries also have their own path dependencies – specific configurations of historical, cultural social and economic circumstances which continue to shape services. Against this backdrop of service evolution, international interest has re-emerged in developing social models of mental health care as a countervailing response to medical hegemony in shaping policy and services. Although, as indicated above, social approaches had emerged in the 1960s for antipsychiatry and labelling perspectives, the new interest in social models is profoundly shaped by the emergence in many countries in the 1980s of service user and survivor movements which have challenged expert-based definitions of need and service delivery. This has in particular brought into question the biopsychosocial model that is seen as leaving medical hegemony unchallenged. The chapter gives a brief overview of the European trends in mental health care, reviews some of the emergent social models and concludes with an attempt to delineate the essential core elements of those models.

Convergence or diversity?

Several statements can be made about mental ill health that seem to stand as generalisations which transcend national contexts. It has been calculated that across both developed and developing countries at any point in time, up to 25 per cent of the population will be affected by mental ill health. Around 1–2 per cent of the population will be experiencing the most severe forms of disorder such as schizophrenia or dementia (STAKES, 1999a). These estimates are based on community studies of prevalence; whether individuals become diagnosed and treated for those disorders depends upon their progress through pathways within the services that exist within any country's health system. Goldberg and Huxley's (1980) influential study of the 'careers' of mental health service users found that primary care was the crucial gateway to specialist psychiatric care. Whether individuals were identified as having a mental health problem, and whether they progressed beyond this point, depended very much on the characteristics and predisposition of the general practitioner. Studies in other parts of the world confirm the view that primary care is the critical gateway that allows or hinders access to specialist services (Strathdee and Jenkins, 1996).

Given the universality of many of these epidemiological patterns, and the generalised statements that are made about pathways in health care systems, it might be assumed that different countries would find similar solutions to the challenges they face. In his 1997 analysis of mental health policy in European countries, Goodwin (1997) argued that at a very general level it could indeed be asserted that there was a shift towards 'community care' from institutional care. Echoing the arguments sketched in the introduction to this chapter, he constructs two ideal-type explanations for this, one based on the radical analysis which saw this as a response to the forces of anti-psychiatry, the other as an optimistic 'Whig' view of the progress of medical treatment and the effectiveness of new pharmacological interventions that made possible the management of mental disorder outside the walls of the institution. However, a finer grained analysis of the particular contexts of mental health suggested to him a more complex mix of influences and trends operating differentially in particular countries. Goodwin (1997) relates his analysis to the debates about 'welfare regimes' that have dominated European social policy analysis in the last ten years, based on Esping-Andersen's (1990) seminal work. Though his pre-occupation was with social insurance systems and the degree to which they provide decommodification of labour, that is protection from the vagaries of capitalist labour markets, numerous writers have extended this approach to other fields of social welfare. Also, in more recent formulations of his thesis, Esping-Andersen (1996) has acknowledged the inherent gender bias within his analysis (labour force analysis based primarily on male participation) and has also compared welfare states according to the degree to which they provide defamiliasation, i.e. autonomy from dependence on the family. Goodwin's (1997) view of welfare regimes in relation to mental health policy suggests, like Esping-Andersen, that despite some analytic limitations of the approach, the clustering of European welfare states provides a useful framework for distinguishing national types and levels of mental health care which are essentially ideal-types – liberal, conservative and social democratic.

Liberal

Liberal regimes are identifiable from the priority they give to maintenance of market relationships in the economic and social spheres. The role of the state is as a safety net when the market fails to provide for basic needs; thresholds for entitlement to services will be set at a level that is perceived not to reduce motivation for individuals to provide for themselves. Benefits will typically be means-tested, selective and consequently are often stigmatising. The United States, Britain and Canada would usually be cited as liberal welfare regimes. In terms of the development of mental health services these countries are characterised by relatively early and rapid deinstitutionalisation. Their mental hospitals had reached their peak in numbers by the 1950s and early 1960s. Services became targeted on acute treatment, with longer-term care increasingly shifted to residential care provided outside the health service.

Conservative

The dominant trait of conservative welfare regimes is the maintenance of the status quo in relation to the economic and social order. It is argued that the role of welfare in conservative countries has been to neutralise the effectiveness of the labour movement, particularly its representation by socialist political parties. Where state intervention occurs it will avoid providing levels of service or benefit that do not improve the position of the recipient beyond their previous status. The state will also take care to avoid replacing welfare provision already being provided by civil institutions such as the church or the family. In Esping-Andersen's typology the Conservative welfare regimes include France, Germany, Italy, Belgium and Spain. In terms of mental health policy, Italy is exceptional because of the reforms led by Psichiatria Democratica, but otherwise these countries have been the slowest to deinstitutionalise; they have also been relatively slow and late to develop community-based services, including day centre and domiciliary support, even in Germany. In these countries considerable emphasis has been placed upon the responsibility of families to provide care for people with mental health needs.

Social democratic

Social democratic welfare regimes see social and economic relations as founded upon social contracts. The state provides services and benefits that are universal, relatively generous and tend to be explicitly redistributive. Denmark, Sweden and the Netherlands are examples of social democratic regimes (although the Netherlands has its own welfare trajectory with a high premium placed upon principles of subsidiarity and 'pillarisation', both of which combine to produce a complex arrangement of welfare). In terms of mental health policy, the social democratic regimes (perhaps counter-intuitively) have been late to deinstitution-alise and develop alternative community-based provision. However, following the tardy shift to community provision in the 1970s and 1980s, there has been a more rapid movement towards rights-based service provision, with the state taking lead responsibility for meeting individual need with less reliance upon provision by the family.

As has been instanced in relation to Italy and the Netherlands, the welfare regime approach provides only a broad-brush approach to understanding the differences between countries. It is also to be noted that it is difficult to locate Ireland within the Esping-Andersen typology. Esping-Andersen himself noted that Ireland did not really fit with the conservative countries where Catholic political parties and church influences remained strong (Esping-Andersen, 1990: 53). As Fanning (2004b) has elaborated, Irish welfare organisations, com-pared to typical European Catholic conservative welfare regimes, have been significantly influenced by the ideological legacy of liberalism, and particularly the introduction before independence of a system of state benefits linked to paid employment.

A research study undertaken by STAKES in 1999 of mental health policies in EU member states found considerable diversity between countries and suggested that: 'Understanding national (mental health) policies requires a more detailed study of the original documents, the values backing them, the quality of implementation strategies and also of the wider societal and historical context.' (STAKES, 1999b: 3) A welfare regime analysis also tends to focus upon quantifiable indicators of welfare, a limitation of the approach which tends to bias analytical variables to those which can be quantified from national statistical sources, such as numbers of hospital beds. It offers less insight into the qualitative changes which are taking place and the policy debates which are driving them. It could be argued that the attention given to the trends in numbers of mental health hospital beds and community-based provision (itself a nightmare for the analyst because of the problems of definition and measurement) provides some broad indication of shifts at a national level between medical and social models of provision, the assumption being that services in the community will have a greater social component. This need not necessarily be the case. Goodwin (1997) himself presents data to suggest that, behind the decarceration from mental hospitals, was an explosion of medicalisation of individual need. This is reminiscent of earlier sociological critiques of the 'psychiatrisation' of society (Castel et al., 1982). The proliferation of diagnostic categories across ever wider areas of social behaviour, and the emergence of technologies to 'treat' them, have produced something rather more complicated than a shift to a social model; it has been the redefinition of the relationship between treatment and care, with the increasing separation between resources which are focused on treatment of those with acute need, and the shunting of care onto providers outside the health sector:

> Overall, there has of course been a shift in the second half of the twentieth century from an institutional to a community-based system of mental health provision. But this. . . . represents little more than the administrative façade for the more substantial aspects of this process: an increasing accessibility of treatment facilities in order to address the newly defined and expanded range of service provision as a means of shifting resources from the problems of psychiatric service users to a more specific focus upon the problem of mental illness. (Goodwin, 1997: 111)

Modernising mental health care: the emergence of new social models

The reconfiguration of services and the ideological differences that are associated with them are often conflated as being about a dispute between adherence to a 'social' or 'medical' model of mental health. In many ways this is like other reductionist approaches that translate a complex argument into a false duality between two idealised alternatives. There are few people today who wish to promote the Laingian idea that mental disorder does not exist and is a miasma created by the combined forces of capitalism and wicked psychiatrists, or Szasz's (1961) once influential view that mental illness is a form of malingering and therefore a moral issue. On the other hand, if there is a positive legacy of this intellectual climate it is the lesson that people who are in mental distress have an authentic voice that should be heard and respected. In addition, it has sensitised providers and users of services to the power relationships through which are defined and applied the categories by which some people are defined as well, and others as ill.

Social inclusion and social capital

A recent systematic review of large-scale epidemiological studies in the west has found a consistent relationship between rates of mental illness and indicators of social disadvantage, including low income, education, unemployment and low social status (Fryers et al., 2003). If we take low income or poverty as one example, it is clear that there are a number of correlations with mental disorder, regardless of the specific mechanism that relates the condition of poverty to mental disorder, e.g.:

- Higher rates of suicide
- Lost production by people who are unable to participate in the labour force
- Reduced labour force participation by carers looking after the mentally ill person
- People being unwell while at work
- Financial dependency of the mentally ill person
- Conduct and emotional disorders leading to educational failure, and subsequent unemployment and illness in adult life
- Potentially impaired emotional, cognitive and physical development of the children of mentally ill parents.
- Lack of educational and employment opportunities leading to failure to achieve potential and continuing frustrations in relation to opportunities.

Mental illness can reduce functioning at home, in education or employment, and the restricted life opportunities this produces continue to contribute to poor mental health in an ongoing cycle. This is one example of the interaction between one social variable and mental disorder. There are many others that could be substituted for this. How these interactions can be modelled into an overview of the possible relationships between social factors and well-being can be represented diagrammatically as in figure 1.1. This kind of model derives from social psychology and consequently views social factors as 'inputs' which are then mediated by individual factors such as socio-emotional variables, people's experience of severe life-events and difficulties and the availability and adequacy of their support networks. As was demonstrated in Brown and Harris's (1978) groundbreaking research into the relationship between social factors and depression, severe life-events in combination with low social support can be 'toxic' for the individual (Brown and Harris, 1978). The model also recognises cognitive factors, such as the level of access to information and personal controls, and beliefs and attitudes. For some critics this type of model is still too medical or individualistic in its orientation, though it has the advantage of offering a framework which suggests why some people might be resilient to the effects of social disadvantage, while others are adversely influenced. As Tew has stated in relation to social models generally:

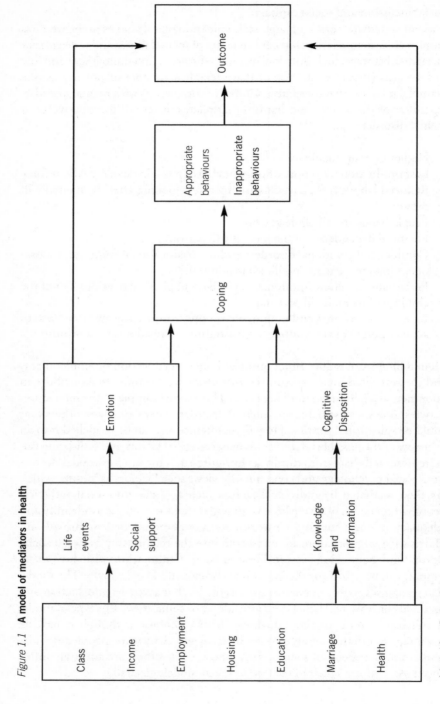

Figure 1.1 **A model of mediators in health**

Adapted from Rutter, Quine and Chesham (1993).

Rather than taking the extreme position that 'mental illness' does not exist, a social model need not rule out the possibility that some people may have greater innate vulnerabilities to particular experiences due to medical, nutritional, genetic or other factors. However, over and above any biological predisposing factors, evidence suggests that a variety of social factors may play a major role in contributing to longer-term vulnerability to breakdown or distress. (Tew, 2002: 147–8)

Increasingly in recent years mental health experts have looked to social inclusion as an analytical framework for conceptualising this relationship between social factors and mental distress, and have gone so far as to argue that social inclusion offers an over-arching framework for understanding the relationship between social factors and mental health (Williams, 2003, Cameron et al., 2003). Social exclusion theory, which originated in continental Europe, asserted that traditional discourses on poverty, exemplified by the British tradition of empirical poverty research, overlooked the multidimensional character of the lives of people who were unable to participate in mainstream social activity because of of their various deprivations. Hills et al. (2002), in attempting to offer a general model of social exclusion, see the individual as surrounded by a series of contexts, from family and locality going outwards in a series of 'onion rings' to the global economy. The key activities in which a citizen should, if they choose, be able to participate are: consumption (the capacity to purchase goods and services); production (participation in economically or socially valuable activities); political engagement (involvement in local or national decision making); social interaction (integration with family, friends and community) (Burchardt et al., 2002: 31).

In fact the mental health literature tends not to be systematic in addressing how mental distress is implicated in these dimensions of social exclusion, but draws on research to show the processes by which people experiencing mental distress are often, through processes of stigmatisation and powerlessness, disadvantaged in terms of consumption, employment, political engagement and social interaction. It can be seen why social inclusion has become a useful form of conceptual shorthand for these effects.

Discussions of social exclusion also merge into the consideration of another influential development in recent social theory, social capital. Putnam (2000) pointed to the apparent decline of social solidarity experienced by people in their communities, the level of engagement they had with networks and civil society and the negative consequences of this. People with mental distress may also be at risk of possessing low levels of social capital, and this appears to be an emerging focus for further empirical research. The theoretical and empirical work that bridges mental health, social inclusion and social capital seems to be part of a resurfacing of interest in approaches linked to community development – another set of intellectual echoes of the 1960s and 1970s. A UK report produced by the King's Fund and the National Institute for Mental Health in England, *Community Renewal and Mental Health*, seeks to identify the working partnerships that can be developed to produce locality-based initiatives to alleviate mental distress and promote well-being (Cameron et al., 2003). This recognises that many of the earlier projects that used community work methods to build alliances with service users and local community groups had become 'squeezed' in the 1990s by a narrower service focus on people experiencing severe mental health problems, while addressing a mental health policy agenda that was increasingly characterised by fears of the challenges that mentally ill people were perceived as making to public safety. This was accompanied by measures that brought people with mental health problems into closer association with areas of high deprivation such as: moving people with mental health problems into social housing projects where social problems were already concentrated; stressors arising from living in areas with poor opportunities for leisure, education and employment which exacerbated individual problems; and the greater likelihood of experiencing poor physical health in deprived areas also exacerbating mental health difficulties. The report's authors identify a range of opportunities arising from schemes such as urban regeneration partnerships that can enhance economic development and social capital development in ways that are inclusive of people with, or vulnerable to, mental health problems.

Disability theory and the service user movement

Much of the political and theoretical impetus for a new social model has emerged from the disability movement and the development of disability theory (Beresford, 2002). It is a significant feature of these developments that, perhaps more than any other area of social theory, this has emerged through 'praxis', the close interaction of political activism and theoretical reflection upon that experience. Key individuals such as Mike Oliver, Colin Barnes and Vic Finkelstein are notable for their own personal commitment to activism as well as to building theory. The departure point is generally given as the manifesto of the Union of the Physically Impaired Against Segregation (UPIAS) first adopted in 1974 (Oliver and Barnes, 1998). This promoted the argument that disability is not a characteristic of the individual, but is a quality of the physical environment that excludes individuals from social and economic participation. At one level this is a simple observation, and yet such is its potency that it has had profound effects on the academic and political discourses concerning disability, and has provided a significant driver in the development of anti-discriminatory legislation. It has also been a catalyst in the development of a self-aware service user movement that demands to be consulted and to be a stakeholder in the development of services. This also extends to the emergence of user-led research in disability and other fields.

Disability theory, which of course has now gone some way beyond the primary definition of disability as environmental exclusion, although identified with movements of physically disabled people, seems to be salient as a generic theory of disability which can be applied to mental health. Barnes and Bowl (2001) have analysed the service user and survivor-led activism as a 'new social movement' with distinct political strategies:

> The aim is not a redistribution of wealth but to gain control over the discourse within which lives are constructed. These transformative rather than redistributive goals affect the nature of the social action within which contemporary movements are engaged. Contemporary social movements adopt a variety of forms of action which are not based in traditional forms of political participation – such as party membership or political participation - but which utilise a range of sub- and counter-cultural strategies such as festivals, the celebration of alternative life styles, consciousness raising and direct action. (Barnes and Bowl, 2002: 136)

The mental health user-led social movements have been identifiable in the United States and Netherlands since the 1970s. Dutch innovations such as the 'clientenbond', a patients' union established in 1971, and the National Council of Patient Advocates established in 1981, have been significant models for groups in other European countries. A study in the UK by Jan Wallcraft (Sainsbury Centre for Mental Health, 2003b) found that indeed many mental health activists consciously saw themselves as part of a broad social movement to empower people who used or had survived the mental health system.

Despite these gains by users and survivors, it is notable that from within 'mainstream' disability theory mental health is not very visible. A 'state of the art' textbook on disability theory contains only two passing references to mental health (Barnes et al., 2002). It seems unfortunate that disability theory offers conceptual ammunition for people working in the mental health field but has not been fully taken on board within the wider disability field as a framework for theory or practice. In an editorial for the *Journal of Mental Health*, Peter Beresford argued for the potential centrality of disability theory as a pillar of a social model of mental health:

> Survivor activists are increasingly considering how such a social model might apply to their situation. There is an interest in developing discussion about the social model of disability to see how it might provide a helpful framework and might need to be adapted for a new 'social model of madness and distress'. (Beresford, 2002: 583)

As Beresford goes on to argue, the framework of disability theory when applied to mental health shifts the taxonomy of the discourse from 'crisis intervention', 'acute episodes' and 'breakdown' towards 'support', 'personal assistance' and 'non-medicalised provision'. The symbolic attainment of this kind of model in the disability field has been the creation of direct payment schemes, now under-pinned in the UK by legislation: this gives money directly to those assessed as having needs who can then directly commission their own package of services. However, the barriers to be overcome in moving to this model of provision are indicated by a Scottish research study that finds that within direct payment schemes people with mental health needs are almost invisible (Ridley and Jones, 2003). Many professionals evidently persist in seeing people in mental distress as inherently unable to make competent choices about their own care.

Quality of life

A further contribution to a new social model of mental health might also be attributed to the emergence of quality of life analysis. For some this may be controversial to bracket with social approaches as much of the development has emerged from within psychiatry and is associated with more positivistic approaches to research and service development. However, the provenance of quality of life analysis is intrinsically connected to the emergence of community-based care as an alternative to institutional provision, and the concern that there should be reliable methodologies for evaluating the relative benefits of different service models to those people who are users of them. Central to quality of life analysis is the measurement of components of quality of life which are non-medical: subjective well-being and satisfaction with different life aspects; objective functioning in social roles; and environmental living conditions (standard of living, social support) (Katschnig, 1997). Key to the methodology of quality of life analysis is eliciting from service users their own perceptions of aspects of their lives which are priorities as targets of change and improvement; often these are not the assumed priorities for psychiatric intervention of compliance with medication and symptom reduction:

> In addition to having specific additional needs for treatment, psychiatric patients are disadvantaged since they usually have fewer resources to cope with life prob-lems, fewer social and cognitive skills and fewer environmental assets, especially money. In many studies of the quality of life of schizophrenic patients in the community, the lack of money is a prominent complaint, probably because it stands for autonomy, which they strive for. (Katschnig, 1997: 11)

In the UK there is now a significant amount of research which has utilised quality of life analysis as a tool for evaluation of social interventions in the lives of people with mental distress (see Huxley, 1997; Oliver et al., 1996):

Quality of life assessment gives social workers a systematic way of assessing in life domains which have meaning to patients and put their views at the centre of service provision and planning. (Huxley, 1997: 137).

Various assessment tools based on QOLA are now available, specifically adapted for use in social and community care contexts.

The recovery model

Also very influential in a number of countries has been a further user-led model, the recovery movement. Onyett (2003) has commented that, in the face of considerable fragmentation between professionals and user-led perspectives, there has been a surprising convergence around 'recovery' as a unifying perspective. Onyett's view is that recovery emerges from a range of theoretical perspectives, although in a wide-ranging review of the recovery literature, Allott and Loganathan (2002) place primacy on the influence of Mary Ellen Copeland as a figurehead in the United States, as well as influential practice developments in New Zealand. Although there is a longstanding recognition in the clinical literature that many people diagnosed with mental distress experience 'spontaneous remission', this is usually portrayed as being an exception to the generally pessimistic prognosis that characterises the discourse. Recovery as an approach to social perspectives in mental health begins from a basic value position that individuals should be empowered to optimise their own well-being and self-direction:

Instead of focussing on symptomatology and relief from symptoms, a recovery approach aims to support an individual in their own personal development, building self-esteem, identity and finding a meaningful role in society. Recovery does not necessarily mean restoration of full functioning without support, including medication; it does mean developing appropriate supports and coping mechanisms to be able to deal with mental health experiences rather than being given supports by mental health services, traditionally known as rehabilitation. (Allott and Longanathan, 2002)

As the authors of this review acknowledge, the evidence-base for the recovery approach is still relatively undeveloped, but there is no doubting its influence as a mobilising ideology for parts of the service-user movement and some professionals.

The Ohio Mental Health Consumer Outcomes Initiative (www.mh. state.oh.us/initiatives/outcomes/outcomes.html) provides an exemplar of how mental health services can adopt a recovery approach, incorporating user-defined outcome measures to evaluate its services. In a break with top-down, clinical approaches to outcome measurement, the initiative utilises an outcome scale developed by user groups over a 16-month period. The domains measured by the scale cover:

- clinical status including the level of symptom distress
- quality of life, the consumer's perspective on their mental health status and its impact on their capacity to experience and enjoy life
- functional status, the ability to manage the basic tasks of daily living
- safety and health including the person's desire not to harm themselves or others
- empowerment

In evaluations of the scale it is claimed that these consumer-defined indicators of the extent to which needs are being met are better predictors of mental health outcomes than conventional clinical outcome scales.

Onyett has commented that the recovery approach has much in common with the 'strengths' approach to case management developed by Rapp and others in the United States (Rapp and Wintersteen, 1989). For instance, that interventions are based on the principle of user self-determination; the recognition that people with severe and enduring mental health problems retain a capacity for change and self-development; that professional involvement should concentrate on strengths rather than pathology; and that the quality of the relationship between service user and care co-ordinator is fundamental. The strengths approach has been influential on both sides of the Atlantic in relation to training, although there must be some questions about whether an approach which is directed towards care *management* can be fully equated with the egalitarian and radical thrust of the recovery approach as articulated by recovery activists.

The social models: essential characteristics and future challenges

Although the development of mental health services in particular countries is shaped by their institutional context, culture and history of welfare, there has been a very broad convergence towards community-based models of care which embrace to varying degrees elements of social models. Inevitably there is a degree of selectivity in instancing particular models, but it has been suggested that social inclusion, disability, quality of life and recovery are all contributory to those developments. They differ in their intellectual provenance, but it might be suggested that they share at least some principles that are core to contemporary social models:

- Many of the problems experienced by people in mental distress are produced by the exclusionary tendencies of social institutions rather than the inherent limitations of those individuals.

- The operation of power is critical in understanding the dynamics of mental health, and inequality is toxic for health and well-being.
- Social inclusion for people in mental distress is multidimensional and includes their position as producers, consumers, participants and social actors.
- Support should be given to people to recover (and exceed) levels of social functioning and inclusion that they have lost.
- Respect should be given to the voices of people who experience mental distress and the variety of their experiences and identities.
- A needs-based and holistic approach to service delivery requires the development of integrated and joined up services, including those led by service users themselves.
- The quality of life desired by people in mental distress is multifaceted and goes beyond the effects of compliance with pharmacological interventions.
- The evaluation of service quality should go beyond professionally defined measures of effectiveness but seek to measure outcomes that have been identified by users of services as important.
- The knowledge base for effective service delivery and professional intervention should be pluralistic rather than positivistic, incorporating findings from user-led research as well as practice-based evidence.
- A unifying value position for the social model is the realisation of autonomy for service users, a concept that goes beyond consumerist conceptions of 'choice' but views the achievement of critical autonomy as a fundamental human need. (Doyal and Gough, 1991; Barnes and Bow, 2001)

For the social models of mental health and their influence upon policy in national contexts, it may be the best of times, it may be the worst of times. As was argued earlier in the chapter, there is a resurgence of interest in the social dimensions of mental well-being that is probably stronger than at any time since the high points of anti- and critical psychiatry. These models emerge from the 'praxis', the interaction of theory and practice, of alliances of service users, practitioners and academics and is particularly grounded in the experience of people living with mental distress that differentiates these models from those earlier movements and intellectual trends. How these models are being expressed and acted upon is shaped, as we have seen, by the national and institutional contexts in which they develop.

So much for the 'best', as for the 'worst' – it is happening at a historical epoch when welfare states in many countries are experiencing retrenchment and restructuring in response to global and regional economic pressures (Pugh and Gould, 2000). These not only constrain the development of services, but they can also add to the very social conditions such as forced migration, unemployment and widening inequality that generate mental health problems. In the UK there are new initiatives which make innovative approaches to social aspects of mental health, such as initiatives to link urban regeneration initiatives with the mental health agenda; at the same time surveys of mental health services show that most National Health Service mental health services struggle to deliver in the face of financial deficit and staff shortages. At the same time the latest movement towards integration of health and social care services, whilst holding out the prospect of seamless and efficient service delivery, also removes the independence from medical services of the professionals who represent the social dimension. Whether 'integration' really means assimilation is not yet clear. Crucially, many of the theoretical and practical developments we have considered happen at the interstices of the welfare state – in voluntary organisations, user-led movements and research centres which are funded outside the mainstream. The survival of these initiatives may be the precondition and barometer of the continuing evolution of social dimensions of mental health policy and practice.

Chapter 2

Mental health in the community

Michael Bergin
Jean Clarke

Introduction

An estimated 450 million people worldwide experience mental illness and/or psychosocial problems; however, only a relatively small minority receive treatment (WHO, 2001a). Mental health is a complex concept and is often perceived with uncertainty, especially in relation to how it is defined. In many parts of the world, mental health and mental illness are not seen as having the same importance as physical health. Principally, this relates to the dominance of a biological framework of understanding health and illness where the embodied sense of self or what Edwards (2001) terms the 'self-project'[1] is not considered. According to Sartorius (1998), the value that individuals, families and communities ascribe to mental health, if improved significantly, could subsequently motivate people to enhance and promote their mental health. Specifically, the concept of mental health needs to be explored and developed within varying contexts and cultures (WHO, 2002a).

This chapter begins with a brief historical overview of mental illness and mental health policy in Ireland. This provides context for an exploration of the key concepts of mental illness, mental health and community mental health. An assessment of the stage of development within current mental health policy is presented. The chapter concludes with a view of the challenges presented by the future, in particular homelessness, equitable resources, stigma and mental health policy. Some propositions for addressing these challenges are offered.

---

1   Self-project is defined as that which is described in the narrative or story of a person. According to Edwards (2001: 104) 'All narratives, by definition, . . . involve social elements, language, culture and . . . appeal to spatio-temporal properties.'

Historical background

Historically, care of the mentally ill reflects a cyclical pattern, ranging from care in the community prior to the nineteenth century, to total institutional care (initially care in the asylum[2]) and currently a return to a community care approach. During the nineteenth century, prior to the development of the asylum system, service provision for the mentally ill in Ireland was essentially cruel in nature; it offered a system of confinement, incarceration and degradation, within jails and houses of industry (Robins, 1986). Oppression prevailed and the mentally ill, referred to as 'lunatics',[3] were not well tolerated within society. During this time it was generally accepted by society that insanity was a moral weakness that necessitated cruel and harsh treatments (Hensey, 1988).

Eighteenth and nineteenth centuries: care in the asylum

Towards the end of the eighteenth century and with increasing accounts of the cruel treatment of the mentally ill, reformers such as Philippe Pinel in Paris and William Tuke in York adopted a more humane approach to care within asylums. They successfully implemented non-restraint methods of care, which brought about a reduction, though not a cessation, in the use of chains to manage behaviour (Repper and Cooney, 1994; Robins, 1986). This approach extended across Europe and America and, in turn, led to provision of specialist professional care within asylums for those labelled as suffering from a mental illness (Saris, 1997). The Lunacy (Ireland) Act 1821 allowed for the construction of district lunatic asylums during the nineteenth century (Walsh, 1987). Indeed, as soon as asylums were completed they were filled. According to Mangen (1985) a diagnosis of insanity during this period would invariably lead to incarceration. At the beginning of the twentieth century, resident figures for asylums represented 0.5% ($n = 16,170$ (1900)), by 1958 it was 0.7% ($n = 21,000$) of the population (Walsh, 1987).[4] Residents included both the mentally ill as well as those suffering from an intellectual disability (otherwise known at that time as 'idiots') (Hensey, 1988). It is important to note that incarceration usually meant confinement without choice and in many circumstances those admitted to asylums were never discharged home to their communities. The asylum system, although

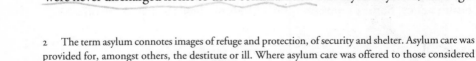

2   The term asylum connotes images of refuge and protection, of security and shelter. Asylum care was provided for, amongst others, the destitute or ill. Where asylum care was offered to those considered insane, this was referred to as the lunatic asylum.

3   The term lunatic, used to describe a person with a mental illness, grew from an association of illness behaviours with the cycle of the moon and the belief that these behaviours or 'lunacy' fluctuated with the phases of the moon.

4   Figures based on estimated population figures for 1900 (3,324.000) and 1958 (2,898,000) (CSO, Ireland).

intended to provide a refuge for those 'suffering' from mental illness, became a system of custodial care, where individuals were separated and segregated from their families and communities, often for a lifetime.

Twentieth century

The nineteenth-century legislation remained operational until the Mental Treatment Act 1945 that established the role of Inspector of Mental Hospitals as well as procedures for voluntary and involuntary admissions to such institutions. This provision was to make the service more acceptable and to improve efficiency (Hensey, 1988). Under this legislation, the Inspector of Mental Hospitals was required to inspect services that provided care for the mentally ill and make recommendations thereon.

Challenging institutional care

In the second half of the twentieth century the writings of Barton (1959) and Goffman (1961) began to problematise the asylum and the practice of institutional care for people with mental illness. Barton (1959) described the process of institutionalisation as feelings of apathy, isolation, loss of interest and a willingness to accept without question, culminating in institutional neurosis. Goffman (1961) in his work *Asylums* highlighted the negative influences of institutional care. Essentially, institutional care was questioned in relation to its ability to offer rehabilitation and the prospect of return to a normal life in the community (Barton, 1959) and there was a movement towards the development of a community-oriented service (at least in the United Kingdom) at this time (Jones et al., 1978). Simultaneously, the introduction of psychotropic medications further advanced the community care approach (Walsh 1987).

Towards a community care approach

In Ireland, movement towards a community care approach to mental illness services began with the appointment by the Minister for Health in 1961 of the Commission of Inquiry on Mental Illness, which reported in 1966. The report recommended the need for change from psychiatric hospitals as the sole centres of care for the mentally ill, to a community-based service (Department of Health, 1966). In addition it recommended the following:

- Integration of psychiatric services into general hospitals
- Rehabilitation for long-stay patients
- Development of outpatient services
- Specialist services for alcoholism and drug addiction, children and adolescents
- Improvement in the education of professional staff in relation to psychiatry
- Amendments to the current legislation to allow for less formal admission procedures to psychiatric hospitals

(Hensey, 1988)

While these recommendations heralded a move away from incarceration and confinement of the mentally ill towards a model of integration, including specialist services for specific groups and specific lifestyle condition, progress was slow. Walsh (1987) and Webb et al. (2002) attribute this to poor economic circumstances and hence financial constraints. However, despite the slow progress in the development of services, the principle of community-oriented care had nonetheless been established. In particular, the need, where possible, to care for someone with a mental illness within their family and within their community was recognised.

Attempts to replace the Mental Treatment Act 1945 with new legislation in the form of the Health (Mental Services) Act 1981 were unsuccessful owing to what Walsh (1987) terms 'technical legal reasons'. Principally, elements of the 1981 Act were considered not to protect the rights of individuals within an international context.[5]

In 1984, the report *The Psychiatric Services: Planning for the Future* was published. It became the main operational framework for the development of the psychiatric services and, in particular, for the development of a comprehensive, community-oriented service, multidisciplinary in nature and integrated within the community (Department of Health, 1984). Noteworthy within this framework was the style of language used – ecological, sociological and moral – and a movement towards a more holistic understanding of caring for people with mental illness.

> [A community-oriented service should] not result in a break with the patient's family, work and other social commitments . . . the level of help and understanding shown to the mentally ill by their family, friends and workmates has a great influence on their recovery.
>
> (Department of Health, 1984: 11)

The emphasis at this time remained on mental illness, however, albeit within a movement towards the provision of care in the community. A shift towards the notion of mental health began following extensive consultation and the publication of the Green Paper on Mental Health (Department of Health. 1992), the White Paper, *A New Mental Health Act* (Department of Health, 1995b), *Guidelines on Good Practice and Quality Assurance in Mental Health Services* (Department of Health and Children, 1998a) and finally the Mental Health Act 2001.

---

5 Formerly there was difficulty reconciling long periods of involuntary detention that existed under the 1945 Mental Treatment Act which were not changed sufficiently under the 1981 Act. This situation was considered to be in contravention of human rights.

Twenty-first century 218

The Mental Health Act 2001 replaced the Mental Treatment Act 1945 and introduced the role of Inspector of Mental Health Services to replace that of Inspector of Mental Hospitals. This new role acknowledged and accommodated the changing location of service provision from hospital-based services to community-focused care. The Mental Health Act 2001 also provided for the establishment of the Mental Health Commission.[6] Principally the responsibility of the Commission is the proper implementation of the 2001 Act and 'To promote, encourage and foster the establishment and maintenance of high standards and good practices in the delivery of mental health services' (Mental Health Act, 2001: 26–7). In addition, it introduced the role of the Inspector of Mental Health Services to replace that of the Inspector of Mental Hospitals. This new role acknowledges and accommodates the changing location of service provision from hospital-based services to community-focused care.

This brief historical overview of social policy in relation to mental health services has traced the movement from asylum care to community-based care as well as to a changed understanding of mental illness. Noteworthy is the change towards the use of the term 'mental health' in legislation: this began in Ireland in the final decades of the last century. Elements of mental illness and mental health need to be considered in order to develop our understanding of mental health in the community.

Understanding mental illness and mental health

Mental illness

Mental illness is viewed primarily as a biological condition and psychiatry as a medical speciality is concerned with the study, diagnosis and treatment of mental illness. While the biomedical model still remains the dominant paradigm for understanding mental health and mental illness (Hannigan and Cutliffe, 2002), some (Pilgrim and Rogers, 1999; Vaillant, 2003) challenge this. The biomedical model[7] principally focuses on the illness without necessarily taking full

6 The Mental Health Commission was established in 2003 and is currently working towards the full implementation of Part 2 of the Mental Health Act 2001. This section of the act deals with involuntary admission to approved centres. It is worth noting the findings of Wells's (2004: 1) study in relation to the implementation of community mental health policy in the UK, which indicated that prioritisation was influenced by the nature of the 'audience' that needed to be satisfied that policy was implemented. Audience within this context did not include service users but rather those within the structures who were monitoring the policy implementation.

7 Recent progress in the decoding of the human genome and in pharmacology appears to be further enhancing the natural sciences contributions to our understanding and treatment of mental illness (Busfield, 2001).

cognisance of the context of the illness or the individuality of the person with the mental illness. For example, people who are diagnosed as depressed may be treated medically, but without any real effort being made to address the circumstances in which they experience their depression.

Since the 1960s there has been dissent with regard to the dominance of the biomedical or illness perspective, most notably by Goffman (1961), Foucault (1961), Szasz (1981) and Scheff (1981). Brown and Harris (1978) argued that mental illness, for example depression, is social in origin. They identified a set of vulnerability factors or circumstances (such as loss, low intimacy, class) that may predispose people to psychiatric illness, thus highlighting the importance of social issues in relation to the aetiology of mental illness. Later, Busfield (1996) articulated the need to acknowledge mental illness within a cultural and social context, as well as a biological framework, emphasising that this may alter over time and place.[8]

Although the biomedical approach has been the dominant paradigm within the mental health field, the sociological perspectives of societal reaction theory, social causation and social constructionism have created new dimensions for conceptualising mental health and mental illness. In particular, social constructionism (Busfield, 2001: ch. 1; Pilgrim and Rogers, 1999: ch. 1) argues that beliefs about health and illness are dependent on a social, cultural and historical context (McCluskey, 1997). The contribution of sociology and the importance of social processes in understanding mental health and disorder are clearly outlined within the literature, and the challenge for the future is to explore 'the interplay of the biological and the social' (Busfield, 2001: 13). Thus contemporary thinking by most mental health professionals suggests a move towards a 'biopsychosocial model' of understanding (Rogers and Pilgrim, 2001).

Mental health

There is no one single universal definition of mental health; indeed much uncertainty surrounds its meaning and interpretation. Whereas mental illness can be defined as the presence of symptoms, Vaillant (2003) informs us that mental health is something more than the absence of symptoms. Yet historically mental health has been viewed either as the absence of mental illness or a state of well-being (Tudor, 1996) and Armstrong (1995) suggests that to most people (lay and professional) mental health implies mental illness while mental health care is care of people with psychiatric illness. Although Trent (1994) agrees that it would be foolish to deny that there is a relationship between

---

8   Both psychiatric classification systems, the Diagnostic and Statistical Manuals for Mental Disorders (DSM) and the International Classification of Diseases (ICD) demonstrate how psychiatric categories are challenged and disputed, and how they tend to appear and disappear over time, for example, homosexuality (Manning, 2001).

mental health and mental illness, the concept mental health needs to be defined within itself and not by its association with some other concept.

Factors that influence a person's mental health can be categorised as individual, interpersonal, social and cultural (Videbeck, 2001). A summary of the attributes that contribute to and influence a person's mental health are considered to be:

- Biological makeup
- Emotional resilience
- Sense of harmony
- Hardiness
- Access to resources
- Sense of belonging
- Level of social support
- Resistance to stress
- Autonomy
- Competence
- Spirituality

(Herron, 1997; McGoran, 1997; Secker, 1998, Vaillant, 2003)

Lay perceptions of mental health have been described in terms of relationships, i.e. 'friendship, love, sharing and support, or the influence of . . . money, . . . independence and optimism . . . justice and fairness' (McGoran, 1997: 257).

Vaillant (2003) presents six models of mental health and suggests that mental health must always be viewed in terms that are 'culturally sensitive and inclusive'. The six models include:

1 Mental health where the ability to work, play and love are emphasised and objectively sought after
2 Mental health as positive psychology with an emphasis on self-efficacy, self–actualisation and humanistic psychology
3 Mental health as maturity with greater maturity reflecting greater mental health
4 Mental health as social–emotional intelligence
5 Mental health as subjective well-being where the person's experiences are happy, contented and desired
6 Mental health as resilience

Mental health thus portrays an image of a person possessing individual autonomy, social competence, coping styles, the capacity to work and to love and who is striving towards self-actualisation. This conceptualisation of mental health could be viewed as being 'reductionist' and deriving primarily from the expert field of psychology (Secker, 1998); it is also idealistic. Notwithstanding these criticisms, the notion of striving towards self-actualisation is compatible with principles of health explored by Seedhouse (1986) and Smith (1981) and suggests the notion of mental health as a process rather than as a static state. It also supports the inclusion of the narrative or story of the individual, that is, the 'self-project' (Edwards, 2001) as central to our understanding of mental health. Vaillant (2003) believes that each model is equally important and one model should not be perceived as being superior. Thus creativity and flexibility in the employment of these models towards enabling our understanding of mental health are critical. This means being open to an understanding of the individual, their culture (Herron 1997, Vaillant, 2003; Videbeck, 2001), social context (Secker, 1998) and community, and defining mental health within this framework of understanding.

The continuum of mental health and mental illness

Trent (1992) argues that the concepts of mental health and mental illness should no longer be perceived along one continuum (see figure 2.1); rather, what is needed is a movement towards an understanding of co-existence, a situation in which mental health and mental illness can occur in the same person at the same time. One way to explain this is to consider the existence of mental health and mental illness along two separate continua. One continuum considers mental health as ranging from minimal mental health/ill health to optimum or maximum mental health, and the second views the attributes of mental illness/disorder that range from mild to severe mental illness (Trent, 1992) (see Figure 2.2). Tudor (1996) suggests that, based on the assumption of two continua, a person who experiences a mental illness may simultaneously experience good mental health, and may also receive some degree of mental health promotion. From this perspective, it is possible to experience a mental illness and simultaneously have a good level of mental health. This is illustrated in the following brief narrative (see Figure 2.3).

Considered within the single continuum of mental health/mental illness (figure 2.1), Paul would be viewed as mentally ill because of his diagnosis of schizophrenia. When viewed within the parallel continua (figure 2.2), Paul when first diagnosed would be considered as having a severe mental illness/disorder with minimal mental health. However, once managed and supported within his illness, and having returned to work and social relationships, his situation along the continua would move towards optimum mental health on the upper bar and mild mental illness/disorder on the lower parallel bar. The advantage of viewing mental health/mental illness within the parallel continua is that it allows the person to simultaneously experience levels of mental health and mental illness disorder. Working from this premise allows intervention for health and illness; it embraces a biopsychosocial model or holistic model of care and avoids labelling.

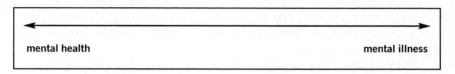

Figure 2.1 **An understanding of mental health/illness along a single continuum**

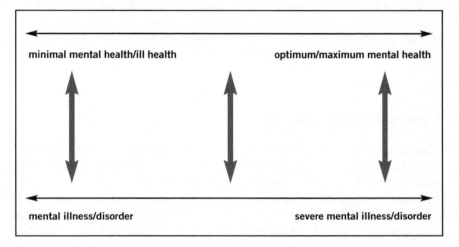

Figure 2.2 **An understanding of mental health/illness along parallel-related continua**

Figure 2.3 **Paul's story**

Paul, 22 years old, has just completed a college education and has started a job in industry as a civil engineer. Paul is fond of sport and plays hurling for his local team; he enjoys the social element of the game as well as a sense of belonging to the local community. He has a wide network of friends and a close relationship with his girlfriend Emma. Paul leaves home to start his new job in the city. Initially he finds the job exciting and challenging but misses the support of home.

Within a couple of months Paul begins to withdraw from the social activity within the office and finds himself increasingly wanting to be on his own. He no longer makes the journey home at weekends to meet with his family and friends. His work colleagues become concerned about Paul and his with-drawal from the activities of work. Meanwhile at home his family are worried about his behaviour. When speaking to him on the telephone, they have noticed that he speaks very negatively about his work colleagues and their suspicious attitude towards him, in particular one colleague who is trying to cause him harm.

When his girlfriend visits for the weekend she persuades Paul to see a doctor who refers him to a psychiatrist. Paul is admitted to hospital and is subsequently diagnosed with schizophrenia. Later, following assessment and treatment he is discharged home, where his treatment continues within the community care services.

Although Paul may return to his original life within the community, fulfil his previous roles (personal, social, work) and enjoy optimal mental health, he may, however, experience periods of minimal mental health or ill-health despite his mental illness being managed. Issues in relation to his work, finances, family and private life, his diagnosis of a mental illness, and how both society and Paul himself perceive the illness, may cause him to experience fear, anxiety, anguish, isolation or distress from time to time.

Community mental health

The development of a community care approach to health care, including mental health, has been greatly influenced by the World Health Organisation's philosophy of Primary Health Care, which is based on the principles of equity, participation, holism, collaboration, health promotion and international co-operation (WHO, 2001a, 1999, 1991, 1978). The focus of the primary health care system is to meet the needs of the individual, family and community through services that are located as close as possible to where people live and work, thus reducing dependence on hospital care. The National Economic and Social Council (NESC, 1987) endorsed the principles of Primary Health Care and more recently the government in its Primary Care Strategy (Department of Health and Children, 2001e: 7) stated:

> Primary care is the appropriate setting to meet 90–95 per cent of all health and personal social service needs. The services and resources available within the primary care setting have the potential to prevent the development of conditions that might later require hospitalisation. They can also facilitate earlier hospital discharge.

Primary care and community-based services
Specifically in relation to mental heath, the Primary Care Strategy advocates the development of a broad focus of services to include:

- Generalist aspects of services for mental health
- Liaison with specialist mental health teams in the community 'to improve integration of care'
- Integration with specialist institutional services

However, in its critique of current services in Ireland the Primary Care Strategy notes the following inadequacies:

- An emphasis on diagnosis and treatment with weak capacity for prevention and rehabilitation
- Secondary care providing many services that are more appropriate to primary care
- Limited availability of many professional groups (e.g. social workers, occupational therapy, physiotherapy, counselling, home help)
- Limited teamwork

(Department of Health and Children, 2001e)

It is worth stressing that during the consultation process leading up to the publication of the *Quality and Fairness* health strategy, 'the needs of people with mental health problems got more attention in submission than other conditions' (Department of Health and Children, 2001f: 18). Specifically respondents highlighted the need for support and treatment in the community. This suggested that current community mental health services were not responding to the needs of the community.

Use of services and the 'revolving door'

There is evidence of a 'revolving door' (Daly and Walsh, 2003) process in relation to current mental health care. In 2001 there were 24,446 admissions to Irish psychiatric hospitals and units, of which 7,301 were first time admissions. Re-admissions accounted for 70 per cent of all admissions, a trend evident since the 1980s. This level of dependence on in-patient hospital facilities has prompted the Mental Health Commission (2003: 5–6) to acknowledge disillusionment in relation to the mental health services, in particular that the service is overly dependent on hospital beds and medication with a lack of 'community mental health teams with true multidisciplinary capacities'.

Where community care mental health services do exist evidence suggests that they are not being used appropriately. A study by Hickey et al. (2003: 5) of psychiatric day care in two health board areas in Ireland found that many 'day hospitals were not operating as alternatives or complements to acute care'. In addition the study concluded that:

- A significant number of patients were attending a day hospital inappropriately, which could partially be due to the lack of day centre provision.
- Services provided were not generally addressing the needs of the acute mentally ill.
- There was evidence that a 'comprehensive range of treatments' were not available.

(Hickey et al., 2003)

One explanation for the difficulties in achieving optimal mental health services within what are termed 'psychiatric day care' facilities is found in the Inspector of Mental Hospitals report of the psychiatric services for 2002. It articulates that many service providers, including 'clinicians', were doubtful as to the functions and purpose of day hospitals (Department of Health and Children, 2003d). The need for education and training for health professionals in relation to mental health and mental illness is viewed as a quality of care initiative; as is the need for 'retaining people in acute care for as long as they need to be there' as well as putting in place structured preparation for discharge planning to aftercare programmes (Department of Health and Children, 2001f: 97).

Voluntary services

There are a number of voluntary organisations in Ireland that promote positive attitudes to mental health and provide a broad range of services to people and their families who experience mental illness. Mental Health Ireland, Aware, Schizophrenia Ireland, Grow, Out and About (phobias), Samaritans, Alcoholics Anonymous, Bodywhys (eating disorders), the Alzheimer Society of Ireland and the Network of Rape Crisis Centres are among some of the major voluntary organisations. In recent years, many of them have developed an 'interagency' working approach in the area of mental health, for example, Alliance for Mental Health, the South Eastern Region in association with their local health board. Their aims are to create awareness and information about services available and to promote the public's knowledge of mental health and mental illness. Their contribution to the work of the statutory services is highlighted by one particular group of mental health professionals (community mental health nurses) whose responses indicate that voluntary organisations play a pivotal role in providing mental health care in the community (Bergin, 1998).

International perspective

The situation with regard to services in Ireland is worth viewing within an international context where the process of deinstitutionalisation to community mental health services has progressed at varying levels. Why this is so is explained by the availability of financial resources and the degree of social acceptance (of non-institutional care), which can vary from country to country, and within countries. Furthermore, in some countries with advanced community-based systems of care they are facing a new challenge; the provision of appropriate housing and vocational / employment facilities for people with mental health problems (Fakhoury and Priebe, 2002). Professional resistance to change is also viewed as a reason for the lack of progress in community-based services within both Western Europe and Canada (Goodwin, 1997).

Irish perspective

In Ireland, similar challenges have been identified since the beginning of deinstitutionalisation including: varying degrees of hostility by 'professionals and other bodies' to the implementation of a community-based model of care; homelessness; and inflexible service systems (Walsh, 1987). Where community-based services have been developed, there is some evidence to suggest that they reflect a transfer of the institutionalised medical model of care to the community setting (Bergin, 1998). More recently, the Inspector of Mental Hospitals Report (Department of Health and Children, 2003d) indicates a continuing lack of understanding of the benefits of community care and at the same time some degree of reluctance to engage with it.

Amnesty International (2003: 19) describes Ireland's deinstitutionalisation policy and practice as being 'uncoordinated, piecemeal and *ad-hoc*'. Research-based studies exploring the efficacy of Irish mental health services are limited (Webb et al., 2002), except for the annual reports from the Inspector of Mental Hospitals and the Health Research Board. There is, however, some research evidence to suggest that the services are meeting the clinical and social needs of people suffering from chronic schizophrenia (Keogh et al., 2003).

A closer look at the challenges presented here in Ireland suggests the need for training and development programmes for both professional and community groups to help them to shift their thinking and acceptance towards a more individual and community-centred model of care. There is also a need for research into the implementation of mental health policy, both strategically and at a practice level.

Challenges for the future

There are a number of challenges confronting the Irish mental health services, some of which have already been outlined, such as clarifying and broadening our understanding of the concepts 'mental health' and 'mental illness', the 'revolving door' phenomenon, research, and the full implementation of the Mental Health Act 2001. Other challenges include: the provision of adequate funding and resources; ensuring that services are based on equity and determined by the needs of communities; responding to the needs of those with mental health problems who are homeless; ensuring the appropriate development of child and adolescent services, older people services, gender sensitive services; addressing the issues of stigma, suicide prevention and provision of mental health care for a changing population. While it is not possible to explore all these issues within this chapter, four areas that are particularly relevant to any discourse on mental health in the community will be considered briefly: homelessness, equitable distribution of resources, stigma and mental health policy development.

Homelessness

The Dublin Simon Community Annual Report 2002–3 indicates that 22 per cent of people in contact with their services have mental health difficulties, such as depression and schizophrenia. They suggest that a lack of appropriate mental health services is resulting in an increase of unmet needs. Homelessness and mental health problems are extensively studied throughout the Western World (Goodwin, 1997). It is acknowledged that the problem of homeless people with mental health difficulties exists, and presents difficulties for community care. However, evidence suggests that it is not a consequence of the closing down of psychiatric hospitals (Leff, 2001). Homelessness is one of the principal concerns for those with a mental illness and is compounded by the lack of provision by local housing authorities of housing for the mentally ill and the difficulty in obtaining community accommodation owing to the supply and cost factors. This problem needs to be addressed at a number of levels, i.e. the provision of housing and the delivery of collaborative accessible and relevant services, both statutory and voluntary (Department of Health and Children, 2003d). For further discussion of the interconnectedness of mental illness and homelessness, see chapter 12.

Equitable distribution of resources

It is estimated that four of the ten most common causes of disability worldwide are attributed to mental illnesses; however, the mental health budgets of most countries are less than one per cent of their total expenditure on health (WHO, 2001a). This disproportionate relationship is evident in Ireland with the mental health services receiving seven per cent of the health budget in 2003, a decrease from 10.6 per cent in 1990 (Mental Health Commission, 2003). The *Health Strategy* (Department of Health and Children, 2001b) and the philosophy of Primary Health Care advocate provision of a health service based on need and equity. A study by the Irish Psychiatric Association (2003) stated that clinical resources within the Irish mental health services are overstretched and not equitably distributed to areas of greatest need.

Stigma

Stigma and discrimination in relation to mental illness remain a challenge, with many negative and distorted beliefs surrounding mental illness still prevailing in society (Crisp et al., 2000; Social Exclusion Unit, 2004). Stigma conveys a person's social identity as being different which may discredit and devalue that person within their community (Arboledo-Florez, 2001) often leading to their social exclusion. Stigma and discrimination continue to be an obstacle throughout Europe (both east and west) and are hindering reintegration into society and early interventions for those experiencing mental illness (Rutz, 2001). Addressing centuries of stigma and discrimination can be achieved only through the empowerment of communities to understanding the true nature of mental illness and its effects on the individual, family and society (Arboledo-Florez, 2001). The promotion of mental health as a distinct and separate phenomenon, albeit inextricably linked to mental ill-health and mental illness, may dispel ambiguity surrounding mental health and mental illness in the community and its associated stigma.

Developing mental health policy
Contemporary mental health policy in most developed countries is described as being 'highly ambiguous', with policies encompassing and exercising control over mental illness and its treatment, and the promotion of a greater sense of well-being (Rogers and Pilgrim, 2001). The process of developing mental health policies should include communities, families and consumers, reflecting a Primary Health Care approach in developing services that meet the needs of the community and not merely the agenda for professionals (WHO, 2001a). Mental health policy also requires a more informed knowledge base (Conlon, 1999).

Conclusion

This chapter has traced briefly the historical background to mental health policy in Ireland, specifically emphasising the move from an asylum model of care to a community-based approach. The provision of care for the mentally ill has changed substantially over the last number of decades with the primary locus of care now being the community. This has allowed for a considerable reduction in long-stay inpatient numbers though the level of readmission – or the so-called revolving door – needs to be addressed.

Changes in policy have been accompanied by changes in language from 'mental illness' to 'mental health' prompted by the sociological and philosophical debate and a move away from a biomedical model to a biopsychosocial or holistic model of understanding.

Important challenges facing mental health care in Ireland are: addressing the issues of homelessness; ensuring increased resources for the sector along with equitable distribution of available resources; dealing with the stigma associated with mental illness; and the development of a comprehensive and enlightened mental health policy.

Recommended reading
Kelly, B. D. (2004) 'Mental health policy in Ireland 1984–2004: theory, overview and future directions', *Irish Journal of Psychological Medicine.* 61–8. **vol?**
Pilgrim, D. and Rogers, A. (1999) *A Sociology of Mental Health and Illness.* Buckingham: Open University Press.

Robins, J. (1986) *Fools and Mad: A History of the Insane in Ireland.* Dublin: IPA.

Saris, A. J. (1997) 'The asylum in Ireland: a brief institutional history and some local effects', pp. 208–23 in Cleary A. and Treacy, M. P. (eds), *The Sociology of Health and Illness in Ireland.* Dublin: UCD Press.

Webb, M., McClelland, R. and Mock, G. (2002) 'Psychiatric services in Ireland: North and South', *Irish Journal of Psychological Medicine* 19 (1): 21–6.

WHO (2001a) *The World Health Report 2001 Mental Health: New Understanding, New Hope.* Geneva: WHO.

Chapter 3

Mental health and the workplace

Pauline Conroy

Introduction

Between one in four and one in five of the Irish population will be affected by a mental health issue according to the Mental Health Commission (2003: p.18). This amounts to about 700,000 people. Quite apart from the distress experienced by individuals, the loss to the economy in productive capacity foregone is huge and eats into economic growth. In this sense, mental health has a direct impact on employment and the economy.

The relationship between mental health/disability and employment is complex. The predominance of medical models of disability within the field of mental health often deprives those with a mental disability of the status of being viewed as people with a disability. They are viewed as people with an illness rather than as people who experience living with a disability or in a disabling environment. This segmentation or segregation of people with mental disabilities to a space outside the category of disability continues in the current health strategy. Strategies for 'people with disabilities' are separated from 'mental health'. No rationale is provided for this separation (Department of Health and Children, 2001: 141–8). This is not just an Irish phenomenon. A recent European study of attitudes to a wide range of forms of disability, excluded mental disability (European Commission, 2001: 57).

The environment of employment in the western world is itself becoming ever more stressful. With regard to health and safety at work, increasing numbers of those employed complain of stress or alienation from the production process (European Commission, 2002: 79). This has a price in that work-related health problems and accidents at work are now costing about 3–4 per cent of European GNP. In the USA, estimates put the cost of national spending on depression at between $30 billion and $44 billion a year (ILO, 2000). Mental disabilities can also impose a heavy burden in terms of social exclusion, stigmatisation and economic costs for those with mental health difficulties and their families (Department for International Development, 2000: 7).

Despite the costs involved, it is only in the latter part of the twentieth century that the issues facing people with mental health problems or disabilities began to be addressed in an employment framework. Some of the interest in employment has arisen from the gradual closure of large hospital and asylum institutions and the accompanying push to treat mental health problems outside a medicalised environment. The social model of disability has focused more attention on employment discrimination and the segregation of people with disabilities from active labour market participation. In this process, organisations of people with disabilities have insisted on the rights of disabled people to equal treatment and defined discrimination as fundamentally wrong (Gogarty, 1998: 4).

Problems and difficulties in the field of mental health can vary in gravity like any other form of disability. Mental health problems can be short-term or enduring, gravely significant as an impairment or a mild and passing stressful episode. Work, in itself, is not intrinsically emancipatory or therapeutic. Some workplace circumstances are in themselves problematic for mental health such as increasing automation, redundancy, atypical employment, rapid turnover of staff, strains in inter-employee relations, intensified competition, harassment, long hours and demands for more responsive workforces (ILO, 2000). These conditions, separately or in combination, can make a workplace hazardous and unsafe from a mental health perspective.

Anti-discrimination legislation

The employment of people with a disability, including mental health disabilities, is protected by non-discrimination law in Ireland. Discrimination in employment against employees with mental health difficulties has been prohibited since 1998 under the Employment Equality Act. The Act prohibits discrimination on nine grounds, including disability, which is defined quite precisely in Section 2 (1) of the Act. Section 2 (1) (e) defines a mental health disability as:

> a condition, illness or disease which affects a person's thought processes, perception of reality, emotions or judgement or which results in disturbed behaviour.

The definition is almost the same as that used in the Mental Health Act 2001, where in Section 3 (2) mental illness is defined as:

> a state of mind of a person which affects the person's thinking, perceiving, emotion or judgement and which seriously impairs the mental function of the person to the extent that he or she requires care or other medical treatment in his or her own interest or in the interest of other persons.

The Employment Equality Act 1998 prohibits discrimination which exists in the present, or which previously existed or which may exist in the future or which is attributed to a person. In this way, discrimination against a person who is (wrongly) believed to have mental health problems comes within the non-discrimination scope of the Act. Employee personal file records of a person being in treatment for mental illness in the past are brought within the scope of the Act, as are employee absences from work, which might or might not be due to a mental health difficulty. The Employment Equality Act is wide in its scope and definitions for providing employment protection for persons with a mental disability.

The definition of disability used in the Employment Equality Act reflects a medical model of disability, which focuses on the impairment rather than on the relationship between the person with a disability and her/his environment. Definitions used by the World Health Organisation or the Commission on the Status of People with Disabilities rely on definitions that stress impairments which impact on participation in society or have the effect of restricting participation (Conroy and Fanagan, 2001: 16).

This latter form of definition was used by the Central Statistics Office in Census 2002 to make an estimate of the numbers of people with disabilities in Ireland. Question 15 of the Census asked whether an individual had one of a number of physical, mental or emotional conditions lasting six months or more that made it difficult to perform certain activities. The conditions were:

1 Learning, remembering or concentrating (mental disability)
2 Dressing, bathing or getting around inside the home (self-care disability)
3 Going outside the home alone to shop or visit a doctor's office (going outside the home disability)
4 Working at a job or business (employment disability)

The Irish Census definition resembles that used for defining impairments by the United States Census Office (United States General Accounting Office, 2002: 30) including:

• Mental or emotional condition that seriously interfered with everyday activities, including frequently depressed or anxious, trouble getting along with others, trouble concentrating or trouble coping with day-to-day stress
• A condition that limited the ability to work, including around the house
• A condition that made it difficult to work at a job or business

The scope of the concept of employment in the Employment Equality Act 1998 is widely defined and includes job advertisements, vocational training for employment, apprenticeships, employment agencies, recruitment to jobs, promotion and treatment in the workplace. Section 16 (3) (b) of the Act obliges employers to do all that is 'reasonable to accommodate the needs' of employees with disabilities. This can be done by the provision of special treatment or facilities (Section 16 (3) (a)).

The Employment Equality Act 1998 was amended by the Equality Act 2004. Among the amendments of 2004 was a change in the obligation of employers vis-à-vis employees with a disability. The intention was to make the 1998 Act consistent with a new European Union Directive on non-discrimination in employment and occupation (European Union, 2000). The section of the 1998 Act referring to employers making accommodations for employees with a disability up to the level of a nominal cost to the employer was replaced. The Equality Act 2004 obliges employers to make as many adjustments or as much accommodation as long as they do not constitute an undue burden or hardship on the employer. Such a cost/burden would vary from employer to employer, unlike 'nominal cost', which could carry connotations of a standardised amount of expenditure.

The Employment Equality Act provisions in relation to disability confer a statutory obligation on all employers in Ireland to facilitate vocational trainees, apprentices, employees and job seekers with disabilities, including mental disabilities. Employers have no choice but to comply with the law. The intention of the legislation is that job seekers and employees with a range of different disabilities can compete on an even playing field with job seekers and employees with no disability.

Individual employees, who believe they have experienced discrimination in employment, can present the circumstances of their cases to the Equality Authority. The Equality Authority has the power to advance cases to the Equality Tribunal, which makes judicial determinations as to whether discrimination has occurred. Up to 2003, just a few cases of discrimination on disability grounds had been heard by the Equality Tribunal. The majority involved allegations of discrimination by individuals with mobility or other sensory or physical impairments. In the absence of a spread of cases arising from judgements on a wide range of disabilities, it is difficult from restricted case law to know what types of mental disability would constitute a disability under the 1998 Employment Equality Act/Equality Act 2004.

In the United States, some mental disabilities do not count as grounds for discrimination under the Americans with Disabilities Act 1990 (ILO, 2001: 11). These are:

- Compulsive gambling
- Kleptomania
- Pyromania
- Psychoactive substance abuse disorders resulting from illegal use of drugs

- Transvestism
- Transsexualism
- Paedophilia
- Exhibitionism
- Voyeurism
- Gender identity disorders
- Some sexual behaviour disorders

Under American legislation, the fact that a person experiences an impairment or even employment discrimination, does not automatically confer legal employment protection on him or her if it arises in the context of one of the disorders listed above.

The Employment Equality Act 1998 has not been widely used by employees with a mental health difficulty. No cases concerning mental health are recorded by the Office of Director of Equality Investigations for the years 2002 and 2003 (ODEI, 2003). While other forms of disability discrimination – for physical and intellectual disability – have been the subject of cases of non-discrimination, mental health/illness issues have attracted no complaints. This may be due to the relatively small numbers of people in employment with mental health problems.

Labour market outsiders

Employment is increasingly the gateway to the benefits of citizenship. Employment supplies social interaction, social status, the opportunity to obtain a mortgage to buy a house; it provides the income for savings and pensions and the opportunity to live at a minimum level of wellbeing. Having a job frequently supplies a circle of friends and colleagues as well as a daily source of information about everyday life. People with mental health problems and disorders are disproportionately outside the labour market of employment, indeed outside the labour force entirely and condemned to the double isolation of mental illness and workforce exclusion.

While new technologies and flexible family friendly production systems may undoubtedly bring employment closer and within the reach of many with disabilities, this is not the case for those with mental disability. Indeed it may be that employment is increasingly difficult for employees with a mental health disability. While in the nineteenth and most of the twentieth centuries an 'able body' was an essential prerequisite for work and a non-disabled status, 'in the world of the twenty-first century an "able mind" may be far more important' (Barnes, 2000: 447).

This insightful observation by Barnes is a salutary reminder that many facets of the modern economy place employment outside the reach of those with a mental illness/disability. The knowledge economy with its emphasis on learning and psychological attainment, team systems of working in interdependent units, just-in-time production systems and the accompanying pressures and interpersonal skills expected of front line staff working with the public, can be enormous obstacles to employees with mental health problems. As well as the stressful pace of many modern working patterns, employees face so many minor landmines waylaying them on their winding itinerary to inclusion and integration in the workforce.

Mental health and the Irish labour market

Just over one in ten of all people with a disability in Ireland aged 15 to 64 describe themselves as having a 'mental, nervous or emotional problem'. These 28,400 people make up one per cent of the total working-age population. These new facts about mental health difficulties in the labour force are revealed by the Central Statistics Office's Quarterly National Household Survey of 2002 and 2004 (CSO, 2002; 2004b). The one per cent figure is based on people's self-definition and may be greater or less than other methods of measurement using hospital admissions or health service patient statistics. The classification in use in the QNHS includes persons with a mental health problem in the same category as persons with an intellectual disability. What is clear is that 28,400 young people and adults considered their difficulties to be of sufficient gravity that they would describe them as disabling.

From the Central Statistics Office data a picture emerges of the adults and young people with mental health/intellectual disabilities in 2002 and 2004. Such an adult is more likely to be male than female and to be living in Dublin in just under one third of cases. This is consistent with population concentrations in Ireland, but tells us only about current residence and not county of origin. In terms of age, the picture is mixed, with some 43 per cent older, aged 45 to 64 years, and ten per cent are young, aged 15 to 24 years.

The personal circumstances of adults with a mental, nervous, emotional difficulty or intellectual disability are very different from the rest of the population. The overwhelming majority – 82 per cent – are alone, being single, or separated or widowed. This compares with 48 per cent of all people with a disability. The sense of isolation and aloneness that accompanies many forms of mental illness is reproduced in the recorded living arrangements of people with such disabilities in Ireland. This has huge implications for services for people with long standing mental health or intellectual disabilities. Not only do they live alone but also, combined with an absence from the labour force, many live without human interaction.

The great majority of adults and young people in this category are not economically active in the labour force. This means they are neither at work, unemployed nor seeking work. If we add to this proportion those who are unemployed, the non-economically active segment rises to 94.6 per cent of all young people and adults with mental health or intellectual difficulties. Thus the employment rate of persons with a non-physical, non-sensory difficulty is extraordinarily low – considerably lower than that of disabled adults in Ireland as a whole (37 per cent, 2004) or the general adult population of Ireland of the same age (64 per cent, 2004).

Adults and young people with a mental health disability are a minority within a minority in the labour force. The employment rate of adults with a mental disability was startlingly low in 2002 and 2004. In the absence of large-scale studies one may only speculate as to the underlying causes for this remoteness from the labour force and the labour market. Some of the reasons may be related to:

- Prejudice and discrimination in the employment environment
- Belief that employment is incompatible with their condition
- Belief among professionals that disabilities of gravity are incompatible with work
- Historical pattern of labour force exit among persons with mental health or intellectual difficulties
- Difficulties in taking steps to return to work among those who exit the workforce due to a mental health problem
- Insufficient programmes of supports to enable people with mental health disabilities to stay at work/make the transition back to work

Just 4,300 of the 30,000 adults with mental health/intellectual disabilities are employees or are on special schemes. In terms of working hours, four out of ten describe themselves as part-time. Indeed, the average working hours of those with mental health disabilities and intellectual disabilities are 29.5 hours a week, compared with 35 hours for all adults with a disability. Thus employees with mental health problems are more likely to be working reduced hours compared with people with other forms of disability or the working population at large.

The low percentages of persons with a 'mental/emotional or nervous' problem in paid employment are remarkably so in that these low employment rates occurred during a time of labour shortages (FÁS, 2003). In a period of almost full employment, during which labour shortages were creating a demand for migrant workers, adults and young people with disabilities remained remote from the labour market. A significant proportion of those in the category of mental health or intellectual disabilities have self-adjusted their circumstances by occupying atypical forms of employment (shorter hours, part-time work, special schemes).

Anecdotal evidence from service providers would indicate that Community Employment Schemes provide a form of employment, which is adapted to the needs of people with a mental health disability. The schemes are locally based in familiar neighbourhoods, are part-time and have supportive supervision in a low-key environment. The Community Employment Schemes were reviewed during 2003 and were threatened with cuts in the number of eligible partici-pants in 2004 (Dooley, 2003: 3) which may be reversed in 2005. Community Employment Schemes were designed as supports to long-term unemployed persons. The schemes were quickly identified as suitable for people with mental health disabilities who entered them with support from a wide range of com-munity, voluntary and not-for-profit bodies.

Stigma and disclosure at work

Attitudes towards people with a mental health disability may be changing but stigma remains in relation to mental health disability. This was one of the findings of the 2002 study of the National Disability Authority (NDA, 2002: 44). The study asked whether respondents thought that people with a mental health disability should have the same opportunities for employment as everyone else. Forty-five per cent of respondents either did not know or considered that they should not have the same rights as others. The same study found that more than half the respondents would be uncomfortable about people with a mental health problem living in their neighbourhood, four out of ten respondents believed people with a mental health problem should not have children, and two in every ten believed that people with a mental health disability did not have the same rights to fulfilling relationships as everyone else. The NDA study exposed extensive prejudice against people with a mental health disability compared with people with other forms of disability involving physical, sensory or intellectual impairments.

A 2002 study of mental health service users, reported that 31 per cent of service users in the Western Health Board region had experienced discrimi-nation in employment (Brosnan et al., 2002: 91). Some 62 per cent reported losing their job as a result of mental illness, while others had to change jobs because of it. To proceed successfully with a case of employment discrimination, employees would usually have had to disclose that they had a mental illness or difficulty, so that the employer could respond appropriately in the event of a workplace difficulty arising. Many employees in Ireland with a mental ill-ness do not in fact disclose their illness to their employer for fear of stigma or discrimination. Those who do disclose are usually in employment in state and semi-state jobs (McLoughlin and McKeon, 1995). Fears of stigma are real and not imagined. Almost a quarter of people asked whether they would employ someone who suffered from depression answered in the negative (McKeon, 1999: 5).

A UK study reported that 46 per cent of employees would disclose a mental health problem to their line manager. Employees anticipated that managers would be understanding, but only two per cent believed they could supply practical support (Diffley, 2003: 7). This was a very realistic estimation on the part of employees. The same study found that over half of line managers felt they did not have adequate information as to how to manage people with mental health problems. Only four per cent of managers knew exactly how to handle the problem using policies and procedures in place. The implication of the study is that disclosure will not automatically generate a helpful response at work.

To bridge the knowledge and information gap, the UK Department of Health prepared a line managers' resource pack (Mind Out for Mental Health, 2003) or practical guide to supporting and managing mental health in the workplace for distribution during 2003. This interesting initiative is directed not at health professionals or families of the mentally ill, but at workplace managers who encounter mental health problems among employees but have no professional background or training in the subject.

Staying at work

Many forms of untreated mental health problems can have an impact on work performance. Depression or heightened anxiety are conditions that can impair work functioning. Symptoms of anxiety and depression can coexist and together interfere with job performance. This can take the form of tiredness, lack of motivation, poor concentration, forgetfulness, poor timekeeping and attendance Some occupations appear to be at a high risk for developing anxiety and depression, in particular where the workers have responsibility for others, such as managers, teachers, social workers and health workers. However, by virtue of their responsibilities, people in these occupational groups can also represent a health and safety risk in the workplace (Haslam et al., 2003: 74). Other mental health conditions pose specific difficulties for workforce integration on a permanent or temporary basis. This is the case for some forms of schizophrenia on a long-term basis and for unstable forms of bipolar disorder on a periodic basis.

In some employment, extensive and repeated use of sick leave and absence can constitute a barrier to promotion and can lead eventually to dismissal. An employee who cannot attend work regularly or for prolonged periods can be regarded in certain circumstances as incapable of fulfilling his or her contract of employment. The Employment Appeals Tribunal would normally expect a period of 12 to 18 months to have elapsed before an employer dismissed an employee for absence. During this time, the employer would be expected to have received medical reports on the employee's fitness to work, to have monitored absences, to have issued written warnings and to have a prognosis of when the employee is likely, if ever, to regain a fitness to return to work.

An employee who is recovering from a mental illness or disability may want to return to work with altered working conditions. This is a sensitive area. Employers are obliged to take reasonable steps to accommodate employees with disabilities, so long as this does not constitute a disproportionate burden on the company or public service body (Waddington and Hendriks, 2002). Nobody knows what a reasonable accommodation in such circumstances could be, since there is not yet any case law in this area from the Office of Director of Equality Investigations. What is clear is that the employee does not have the right to seek employment in a different job with the same firm or body. Reasonable accommodation is widely understood to be operational only in relation to the core or essential functions of a job for which the job holder is competent, capable and otherwise available.

Many forms of mental illness, such as depression, can be treated successfully nowadays and may only require a limited absence from work. Other mental health problems may require longer clinical care as well as in-depth consideration of workforce reintegration. In these latter instances, pressure to return to work is unhelpful and can be experienced as oppressive. The right of individuals with significant disabilities not to work or to refuse to work is part of the employment framework which reflects the dignity and rights of people with disabilities.

Out of work

Changes in social welfare have made staying out of work increasingly attractive for some people. A person aged 16 to 66 years who is not economically active, is without a job and unable to seek work, because of a long-term mental illness, will be entitled to a Disability Allowance, which is subject to a means test. Disability Allowance in 2003 amounted to €124.80 a week. Since April 2002, it has been possible to earn €120 a week in addition to Disability Allowance, so long as the work is rehabilitative in nature and approved by the Department of Social, Community and Family Affairs. The additional earnings are treated as 'disregarded' in social welfare terms and amount to the equivalent of 17 hours work a week.

Adding together the social welfare payment and the maximum disregard, the total income, earned and unearned, of a person with a substantial disability comes to €244.80 a week. This is equivalent to a 35-hour week on the minimum wage (2004). Besides the Disability Allowance and the disregard, such claimants with a disability are entitled to a Medical Card and free travel. To obtain a monetary value of €244.80 after tax and deductions, a single person would have to earn about €489 gross a week. The combined value of direct and indirect benefits is such that for those with limited education or training, whose opportunities for good earnings are constrained, it is more attractive to stay off the open labour market than to seek an open market low-wage job.

Conclusion

Compared with the working-age population and other people with disabilities, the population who experience a mental health difficulty or mental disability are at a serious disadvantage. Stigma and deep prejudice appear to be part of the cause of their remoteness from economic participation in the life of the country. Frequently living alone on social welfare payments, people with a mental disability are at a high risk of sinking into persistent poverty, social exclusion and homelessness (Crowley, 2003). These factors may explain the absence of people with a mental disability from the statistics of anti-discrimination case law in employment: too few jobholders with a mental disability are in mainstream full-time jobs.

The economic costs of mental illness are high. This is especially the case for depressive illnesses which affect thousands of individuals and is a serious occupational health issue. Fear of disclosure or the consequences of disclosure can prompt workforce withdrawal, depriving firms and the wider economy of the employment benefit of their employees. Thus the management of disability within the workplace has attracted ever-increasing interest among employers and employer bodies globally, with a view to developing job retention strategies for employees who face a mental illness. In the case of mental disability, the importance of the right to work in equalising opportunity between those with and those without a disability must also be accompanied by a decent standard of living for those who exercise the right not to work in the market economy.

The chance to work in a sheltered enterprise could be an opportunity for people with a long-standing mental health disability, when a framework for such enterprises is eventually established by the Department of Enterprise Trade and Employment in 2005. Sheltered Enterprises could be allowed to have preferential treatment in specific public procurement tenders for contract work. Such preferences are allowed under European Union competition law but have not yet been incorporated into Irish law.

Chapter 4

Health promotion and mental health

Iris Elliott

Introduction

Health promotion is a diverse dynamic field, framed by a series of international agreements and fed by multiple disciplines, which has an impact on the health and social well-being of individuals, groups, communities and the whole population. This chapter will begin with an exploration of health promotion in order to locate its sub-field – mental health promotion. Relative to other areas of health promotion, mental health promotion in Ireland and internationally has been marginalised in terms of strategic development, profile, funding and practice.

However, there is an increasing sense that the time of mental health promotion has come. Increasing attention is being given to the mental health field and there are significant international policy levers for action on health – including mental health – promotion, a growing body of international evidence on the effectiveness of mental health promotion interventions, and an expanding infrastructure of national and international organisations and networks that could be resources for Ireland in its development of mental health promotion. The chapter will examine developments in both policy and practice in Ireland in the context of the increasing focus on the importance of health promotion, nationally and internationally. The potential role of mental health promotion and the challenges to maximising its impact will be considered.

There is growing evidence that mental health promotion can:

- improve physical health
- increase emotional resilience, enabling people to survive difficulties and distress
- enhance citizenship, giving people the skills and confidence to adopt meaningful and effective roles in society
- increase productivity
- help to reduce either the incidence or the severity of mental health problems
- reduce the significant costs, to individuals, their families, their employers, the health service and the country as a whole.

(Health Promotion Agency Northern Ireland, 1999)

The *National Health Promotion Strategy* (Department of Health and Children, 2000b) includes a commitment to the strategic development of mental health promotion by 2005, which was reiterated in *Sustaining Progress: Social Partnership Agreement 2003–2005* (Department of the Taoiseach, 2003). The *Review of the National Health Promotion Strategy* was published in 2004 (Department of Health and Children, 2004c). As a result of the health strategy *Quality and Fairness: A Health System for You* (Department of Health and Children, 2001b), an Expert Group on Mental Health Policy was established to deliver the first national policy framework since 1984. Further, the Good Friday Agreement (Government of Ireland, 1998) provides opportunities to develop health promotion on an all-island basis.

Mental health and health promotion: definitions and principles

'Mental health' has been diversely defined, reflecting social and cultural contexts. Conceptions of mental health are dynamic, changing through knowledge and experience exchange. The contested nature of mental health is considered to be the main barrier to the development of sustainable and effective mental health promotion (Herron and Mortimer, 1999), which has led to its relative neglect within health promotion (Tudor, 1996).

Some commentators suggest that mental health promotion cannot proceed without this being resolved (Mauthner et al., 1999). Others advocate pluralism, supporting the co-existence of a multiplicity of definitions, which reflect not an unresolved conceptual problem but an expression of different perspectives on mental health, each with benefits and limitations (Tudor, 1996).

The touchstone document for health promotion is the *Ottawa Charter for Health Promotion* (WHO, 1986a), adopted at the first International Conference on Health Promotion. Subsequent international agreements have built upon this foundation. The Charter defines health promotion as:

> the process of enabling people to increase control over, and to improve, their health. To reach a state of complete physical, mental and social well-being, an individual or group must be able to identify and to realise aspirations, to satisfy needs, and to change or cope with the environment. Health is, therefore, seen as a resource for everyday life, not the objective of living. Health is positive concept emphasising social and personal resources, as well as physical capacities. Therefore, health promotion is not just the responsibility of the health sector, but goes beyond healthy life-styles to well-being. (WHO, 1986)

The Charter goes on to identify the multiple determinants (which it frames as conditions and resources) of health, including social justice and equity. In

Ireland *Quality and Fairness: A Health System for You Health Strategy* acknow-ledges '(s)ocial, economic and environmental factors as the main external or structural determinants of health. At an individual level, factors such as age, sex, hereditary factors and lifestyle choices are important' (Department of Health and Children, 2001b: 10).

Three key influences on mental health were identified by the UK's Health Education Authority in its *Mental Health Promotion Quality Framework* (Health Education Authority, UK, 1997). These are:

1   healthy structures such as the economic, social and cultural framework
2   citizenship, including social support, sense of social integration and inclusion
3   emotional resilience encompassing self-esteem, coping, life skills and sense of control

The *Ottawa Charter for Health Promotion* (WHO, 1986) established the 'five pillars' of health promotion action:

* build healthy public policy
* create supportive environments
* strengthen community action
* develop personal skills
* reorient health services.

In 1998, the World Health Organisation identified seven Principles of Health Promotion to support its strategic development: Empowerment, Participative, Holistic, Inter-sectoral, Equitable, Sustainable, Multi-strategy. The principles outline approaches that include policy development, organisational change, community development, legislation, advocacy, education and communication, in combination with one another. Combined with a holistic and process-based definition of health (as well as acknowledgement of the diverse conditions and resources required for positive health) these areas of action, principles and approaches indicate the substantial scope for health promotion activity at the individual, group, community and population level. The question arises as to how this potential scope is realised in practice.

Tilford et al. (1997) observe that the application of health promotion theories into practice reflects ideological as well as practical considerations. Whilst some commentators suggest that health promotion has shifted its focus from reductionist and individualised models of behavioural change to consider how social structure, processes, relationships and identities impact on health (Raeburn and Rootman 1998), others are less convinced. For example, Ziglio et al. (2000) in their review of health promotion development in Europe note the tendency for health promotion to address health-sector generated, lifestyle and behavioural change programmes, focusing on one health issue or one determinant of health at a time. They comment that 'second-order change, which involves a paradigmatic shift leading to new structures, processes, actions and outcomes, has barely begun to happen' (2000: 145).

The development of mental health promotion internationally

Although mental health promotion can be traced to the Mental Hygiene Movement in Britain in the nineteenth century, contemporary mental health promotion emerged in the 1980s (Mauthner et al., 1999) but has remained marginal within health promotion until recent years. Internationally the publication of the World Health Report 2001, *Mental Health: New Understandings, New Hope* (WHO, 2001a), affirmed the need for action in the mental health field. Prior to this, the publication of the first US Surgeon General report on mental health was another indicator of the attention starting to focus on mental health (US Department of Health and Human Services, 1999).

The World Health Organisation, the European Union and international bodies such as the World Federation of Mental Health and the Global Consortium for the Advancement of Promotion and Prevention in Mental Health have driven strategic action on health promotion. Through its broader remit, the World Health Organisation develops initiatives such as advocating for the inclusion of mental health promotion in mental health law (WHO, 1996b). It has provided an international framework for health promotion by facilitating a series of international agreements and the provision of technical guidance on aspects of health promotion. Key international agreements are:

1986 Ottawa Charter, which provided the foundation for subsequent documents that have built on its five key elements
1988 Adelaide, Australia – developing healthy public policy
1991 Sundsvall, Sweden – creating physical, social and economic environments for health, compatible with sustainable development
1997 Jakarta, Indonesia – identifying professional and technical skills, investing in an infrastructure for health promotion
2000 Mexico City, Mexico (equity in health), leading to the Mexico Ministerial Statement for the Promotion of Health
Verona Initiative (determinants of health, inter-sectoral partnerships) leading to the Verona Benchmark, an investment for health model (Department of Health and Children, 2000b)
2005 Mental Health Declaration for Europe: Facing Challenges, Building Solutions (WHO, 2005b)

There has been considerable health promotion activity in the European Union since the 1990s, sometimes in the context of public health, including policy, research, programme and organisational developments. A timeline of selected milestones is given below:

1992 European Commission established a senior committee for Health Promotion and Education with representation from all Member States. Article 152 Treaty on European Union stated that a high level of human health protection shall be ensured in the definition and implementation of all Community policies and activities.

1995 European Network on Mental Health Policy established.

1996 European Union Health Promotion Programme adopted.

1997 European Network for Health Promotion Agencies established.
Key Concepts for European Mental Health Promotion published.

1999 European Commission Mental Health Indicators Project commenced.
Tampere Conference requested that Member States take action by:
(a) promoting mental health and preventing mental illness
(b) encouraging the exchange of best practice and information
(c) promoting joint projects with other Member States
(d) furthering and supporting research into mental health and its promotion.

1999 European Council Resolution on the Promotion of Mental Health (2000/C86/01) recognised the need for addressing the promotion of mental health by increasing co-operation with applicant countries and inviting the Member States to:
• give due attention to mental health and to strengthen its promotion in their policies
• collect good quality data on mental health and actively share it with other Member States and the Commission
• develop and implement action to promote mental health and prevent mental illness and promote exchange of good practices and joint projects with other Member States
• stimulate and support research on mental health and its promotion, also using the opportunities provided by the Fifth Framework programme of the European Community for research, technological development and demonstration activities. (Council of European Union, 1999)

2000 European Commission's Public Health Action Programme launched
EC Communication on the Health Strategy of the European Community (COM(2000)285 final) adopted.

2003–5 European Commission funded Implementing Mental Health Promotion Action (IMHPA) project delivered.

The themes emerging from these milestones are the importance of:

1 strengthening mental health policy and practice
2 exchanging experiences and expertise
3 stimulating joint research and practice developments on a cross-European basis
4 collaboration between Member States
5 enhancing the value and visibility of mental health in Europe

The European Union's strategic action has included support for international fora to consider the development of a European mental health promotion agenda (STAKES, 1998) and initiatives to develop mental health promotion within a wider public health agenda (Lavikainen et al., 2001), underpinned by a commitment to progressing information sharing and collaboration between Member States. Following the adoption of the European Union Health Promotion Programme in 1996, the European Commission funded mental health projects. These included the Key Concepts Project by the European Network on Mental Health Policy, which focused on the central concepts of and priorities in the promotion of mental health, an assessment of mental health policies in the Member States and indicators of mental health. The Network compiled a report *Framework of Action for Promoting Mental Health in Europe* (European Network, 1997), which informed the identification of the following key areas for preparing the European mental health promotion agenda:

• enhancement of the value and visibility of mental health
• mental health promotion for children and adolescents
• mental health promotion, working life and unemployment
• mental health promotion and the ageing population
• social integration of severely marginalised groups
• development of mental health indicators
• telematics of mental health promotion (STAKES, 1998)

The IMHPA project 2003–5 engaged 21 European countries, four European networks and the World Health Organisation to produce an internet database of programmes, a training manual for health professionals and a policy action plan.

Other significant markers in the development of mental health promotion have included: national research; reviews of activity (Health Promotion Agency Northern Ireland, 1999) and effectiveness (Hodgson and Abbasi, 1995; Tilford et al., 1997; NHS Centre for Reviews and Dissemination, 1997; Friedli, 2003); strategic national statements (Health Education Authority, 1997; Health

Education Board for Scotland, 1998) and policy (Scottish Executive, 2002, 2003); the establishment of the *International Journal of Mental Health Promotion*; and the publication of key texts (Tudor, 1996). However, concerns have been raised regarding the motivation behind this activity. Mauthner et al. (1999) suggest that social policy interest in mental health promotion is driven by psychological morbidity data, the lack of service resources and public demands for care rather than by popular and political desire to promote health.

In Ireland this appears to be supported by reference to the types of data used to underpin mental health and mental health promotion policy. Both national health promotion strategies and the current national health strategy (Department of Health and Children, 2001b) employ data on psychiatric morbidity, suicide, mental hospital admissions and pharmaceutical use. Such data immediately locates mental health within the paradigm of mental illness and mental health service provision.

This narrow approach is reflected in Mauthner et al.'s (1999) findings from their literature review of mental health promotion theory and practice. In contrast to their model of mental health promotion based on the *Ottawa Charter for Health Promotion* which emphasises individual, structural and socio-economic dimensions, they found that 'effective' mental health promotion interventions comprised predominantly individualistic, psychological interventions focusing on coping skills or cognitive processes. This reflects the findings of Ziglio et al. (2000) regarding health promotion in general, discussed on pp. 52–3 above.

Mental health promotion in Ireland

Ireland has had two national health promotion strategies spanning 1995–9, and 2000–5 (Department of Health, 1995a; Department of Health and Children, 2000b). In 2004, the Department of Health and Children published a review of the 2000–5 strategy (2004c).

National Health Promotion Strategy 1995–9
The first Health Promotion Strategy (Department of Health, 1995a) outlined an approach which focused on healthy lifestyles. It included a goal to promote mental health in co-operation with the voluntary mental health bodies and the health boards. It also outlined a number of supporting actions:

• Providing programmes that develop mental and emotional health, self-esteem, personal relationships and coping skills
• Strengthening the individual's basic capacity to make healthy choices and to cope with stressful situations without recourse to behaviours which may damage health

* Continuing support for an intervention study aimed at reducing the pre-valence and cost of para-suicide

During the first national health promotion strategic period, 1995–9, there were significant developments within health promotion, including the establishment of health promotion departments in all health boards, the first nationally representative surveys on lifestyle practices, the inclusion of a commitment to health promotion development in the social partnership agreement and the publication of the Report of the Task Force on Suicide (Department of Health and Children, 1998b).

The health strategy, *Quality and Fairness: A Health System For You* (Department of Health and Children, 2001b) had a timeframe of 7–10 years. With regard to health promotion it referred to the commitments in the *National Health Promotion Strategy 2000–2005* (Department of Health and Children, 2000b) However, mental health is not one of the initiatives profiled from the strategy. In relation to mental health in general, under Objective 4 Specific Quality of Life Issues, Mental Health, the strategy stated that programmes to promote positive attitudes to mental health would be introduced (2001b: 147)

With regard to mental health service development there is a significant commitment in Action 25 which states that 'a new action programme for mental health will be developed . . . A national policy framework for the further modernisation of mental health services, updating planning for the future (1984) will be prepared' (2001: 164). The Expert Group that will deliver this commitment was established in summer 2003 and will report in 2005.

National Health Promotion Strategy 2000–5
The policy framework for mental health promotion is detailed in the *National Health Promotion Strategy 2000–2005* (Department of Health and Children, 2000b). The strategy is organised around topics (of which mental health is the lead), settings and population groups. Specific actions on mental health promotion are given for young people, women, men and older people.

The strategic aim for mental health is 'to promote positive mental health and to contribute to a reduction in the percentage of the population exper-iencing poor mental health' (2000b: 53). Objectives identified in the strategy outline research into models of best practice, the development of a national positive mental health strategy and partnership work on the implementation of the Report of the National Task Force on Suicide (2000b: 53).

The *Review of the National Health Promotion Strategy* (Department of Health and Children, 2004c) highlighted the importance of the new mental health policy as a vehicle to promote positive mental health. It indicated the need to identify and disseminate models of best practice in mental health promotion.

The Good Friday Agreement

The inclusion of health as one of the areas for co-operation identified by the Good Friday Agreement, and the selection of health promotion as one of five health operational areas in which work will be progressed, represent opportunities to progress the development of mental health promotion on an all-island basis.

There has been significant activity in Northern Ireland on mental health promotion including:

- commitment in the Northern Ireland public health strategy, *Investing for Health 2002*, 'to promote mental health and well-being at individual and community level'
- publication of *Promoting Mental Health Strategy and Action Plan 2003–2008*
- establishment by the Northern Ireland Mental Health and Learning Disability Review 2002–5 of a working group on Mental Health Promotion in late 2003
- development of a database of mental health promotion activities
                                       (Health Promotion Agency Northern Ireland, 1999).

The development of all-island mental health promotion can be informed by initiatives such as the study on *Promoting Mental Health and Social Well-being: Cross-Border Opportunities and Challenges* by Barry et al. (2002), which investigated cross-border collaborative mental health promotion practices and examined the compatibility and comparability of mental health and related health data sources. It also identified a number of steps considered necessary for the promotion of best practice in mental health promotion on an all-island basis.

Health promotion organisational structures and resources in Ireland

In 1988, the Health Promotion Unit (HPU) was established in the Department of Health and Children. Under the Government's Strategic Management Initiative, the department will focus on strategic aspects of health policy. At regional level, The Health (Amendment)(no. 3) Act 1996 conferred a statutory obligation on health boards to develop 'health promotion programmes, having regard to the needs of people residing in its functional area and the policies and objectives of the minister in relation to health promotion generally'. Dedicated regional health promotion teams have been established across the country. The Liaison Officers Group, which brings together the Regional Health Promotion Managers and HPU, meets four times a year to discuss and review strategic developments and objectives. These national and regional health promotion resources will be included in the Population Health Divisions, which are being established as a result of a commitment in the national health strategy. An Association of Health Promotion, Ireland, has been established.

Unlike other health promotion topics, there has been no designated mental health promotion officer post in each of the regional health promotion departments. The National Task Force on Suicide (Department of Health and Children, 1998b) led to the appointment of a Suicide Resource Officer in each health board. Some of these took a health promotion approach and a number were re-titled 'mental health promotion officer'. The development of explicit mental health promotion in the regional departments has varied around the country. However, some of the projects and programmes that they have delivered, for example in school and community settings, could be categorised as mental health promotion. Without an audit of mental health promotion activity it is not possible to identify the resources allocated to this area. A health promotion function has been included in the job descriptions of a range of health board personnel. The impact of this inclusion and the resources required to fully operationalise it have not been researched to date. This represents an important health promotion resource in the health service.

Significant mental health promotion activity is generated by the voluntary sector for example by Mental Health Ireland, Schizophrenia Ireland, Aware and Grow. Also, the Health Promoting Hospitals Network, Ireland has established a mental health interest group, which links with that established in the network at European level.

The Department of Health Promotion was established at NUI, Galway to provide education, training and research, with the Chair of Health Promotion supported by the HPU. There are also academic bases for health promotion in Ireland at the University of Limerick, University College Cork and Waterford Institute of Technology.

Mental health promotion activity in Ireland

Tilford et al. (1997) suggest that mental health promotion can address the determinants of mental health separately or in combination by 'reducing the stressor impact of the environment and by increasing the capacity of people to resist stressors' (1997: 51).

Work has begun to identify the level and range of mental health promotion activity on the island of Ireland. Key initiatives have been the establishment of a database of mental health promotion activities in Northern Ireland (Health Promotion Agency Northern Ireland, 1999), the identification and review of projects in the cross-border study conducted by Barry et al. (2002) and the establishment of a database of health promotion activities by the Health Promoting Hospitals Network, Ireland launched in 2003.

Anecdotally there appears to be considerable activity described as mental health promotion. Much of this activity is generated by the voluntary organisations and statutory services in the mental health sector. However, the Health Promoting Hospitals Network indicates mental health promotion activity in general services, often related to the promotion of worker's health for example stress management.

The database compiled by the Northern Ireland Health Promotion Agency in 1999 identified 126 initiatives and categorised them using a system developed by Health Promotion Wales. The 40 collaborative mental health promotion projects across the island of Ireland identified by Barry et al. (2002) in their study underline this diversity. The study noted high levels of projects dealing with suicide prevention and/or depression (23 per cent) and rehabilitative/vocational training (12 per cent). The researchers selected case studies of projects addressing suicide, post-natal depression, positive mental health in rural communities, young people with cancer and their families, and positive mental health.

In addition to activity that is explicitly described as mental health promotion, there are many other activities linked to the broader determinants of mental health that could be considered to have health promotional impacts. The development of Health Impact Assessment (HIA) provides a structured and systematic framework to map out the full range of health consequences of any policy, programme or project, whether these are negative or positive (Elliott, 2001). The current Health Strategy (Department of Health and Children, 2001b) includes a commitment to develop Health Impact Assessment. It is one way in which initiatives can not only be health 'proofed' in order to maximise their positive and minimise their negative impacts on health, but also identified as resources for the promotion of mental health. The *Review of the National Health Promotion Strategy* (Department of Health and Children, 2004c) recommends the progression of a formal health-proofing process in building healthy public policy.

Likely developments and future challenges

Mental health promotion internationally and within Ireland is diversely defined. There is no common agreement as to what constitutes mental health promotion. This can be view as problematic or embraced as indicating an exciting and diverse field in which those within and outside the health sector – the public and professionals – are exploring a range of conceptions of mental health and are evolving practice from these experiences and realities.

In Ireland, as internationally, mental health promotion activity appears to have reached a critical mass. Work towards a mental health promotion strategy, research into the level and range of mental health promotion activity as well as its effectiveness, and the legal basis to develop health promotion on an all-island basis are significant opportunities to move forward.

A consensus is emerging regarding the challenges in progressing this agenda. Action is required in the following areas.

Leadership

The World Health Organisation has identified national governments to be the stewards of mental health (WHO, 2001a). The 2005 Mental Health Declaration for Europe (WHO, 2005b) stated that the promotion of mental health is a priority for the World Health Organisation and its member states and urged the member states, World Health Organisation, European Union and the Council of Europe to take action. Such national leadership must respect and be informed by the wealth of expertise held by the public and health promotion practitioners, researchers and theorists.

Policy and structures

Early research and anecdotal comment indicate that there is a significant level and range of mental health promotion activity in Ireland. To consolidate and accelerate the development of best practice in mental health promotion requires a national policy framework and supportive structures, both organisations and networks. This includes all-island work. In part, this may be progressed by the report of the Expert Group on Mental Health Policy, which is addressing mental health promotion. Such developments would provide the basis for a dedicated budget.

Collaboration

Collaboration includes sharing and disseminating innovative and effective practice, as well as developing new work together. This would involve finding a common language to facilitate communication, while respecting the diversity of mental health promotion practice.

Evaluation

The challenges for effective evaluation in mental health promotion include the identification of:

1   Appropriate evaluation frameworks and research methods that can capture the diversity, creativity and complexity of contemporary practice (Barry et al., 2002)
2   Resources to conduct such evaluation both in terms of finance and staff capacity
3   The timeframe required to yield results (Tilford et al., 1997)

Skills and training

There is a need to build capacity for mental health promotion through training programmes in order to promote quality and vision in practice.

Generating data

The development of mental health promotion requires the collection of both quantitative and qualitative data, and equal value to be given to both. Barry et al. found that 'There is quite limited data on mental health status at a population level or the pattern of differences among different population groups' (2002: 10) and recommended the co-ordination, harmonisation and effective dissemination of data.

Conclusion

The Ottawa Charter for Health Promotion continues to provide the touchstone for this activity. If health promotion is to continue to impact on the mental health of individuals, groups, communities and the whole population, Ireland needs to develop healthy public policies, build healthy communities, develop healthy lifestyles, create supportive environments and reorient health services. For this vision to be realised strategically and equitably, mental health promotion must be resourced with leadership, partnership, debate and finance.

Recommended reading

Barry, M., Friel, S., Dempsey, C., Avalos, G. and Clarke, P. (2002) *Promoting Mental Health and Social Well-being: Cross-Border Opportunities and Challenges.* A Report for the Centre for Cross Border Studies and the Institute of Public Health in Ireland Armagh: Centre for Cross Border Studies and Dublin/Belfast: Institute of Public Health in Ireland.

Tudor, K. (1996) *Mental Health Promotion: Paradigms and Practice.* London and New York: Routledge

WHO (2001a) *The World Health Report 2001 – Mental Health: New Understandings, New Hope.* Geneva: WHO.

WHO with Victoria Health Promotion Foundation and University of Melbourne (2004) *Promoting Mental Health Concepts: Emerging Evidence Practice.* Geneva: WHO.

Chapter 5

Children and mental health

Valerie Richardson

Introduction

It is now recognised that many mental health problems in adolescence and adulthood can and do begin in childhood. Epidemiological studies, while numerous, provide variable rates of recorded prevalence of mental health problems in young people. However, the World Health Organisation (WHO, 2003: 8) has stated that approximately one in five of the world's youth (15 years and younger) suffer from mild to severe disorders and that a large number of these young people remain untreated as diagnostic and treatment services are either minimal or non-existent. Generally cross-cultural comparisons tend to show prevalence rates of child mental health problems as being between 15 and 20 per cent of the age group. (Bird, 1996; Dogra et al., 2002). However, prevalence rates tend to vary according to environmental factors, with higher rates for inner city areas than rural areas and in poorer deprived areas.

This chapter will address the issues concerning mental health problems of children in Ireland. In its submission to the Expert Group on Mental Health Services the Irish College of Psychiatrists defined a mental health problem as 'a disturbance of function in one of the following areas: relationships, mood, behaviour or development of sufficient severity to require professional intervention' (2003c: 41). The definition of a psychiatric disorder is given as 'the presence of a severe and persistent mental health problem/symptom or the co-occurrence of more that one problem that satisfies the criteria for a disorder according to the World Health Organisation (1992) or the American Psychiatric Association (2000)' (Irish College of Psychiatrists, 2003c: 41) Based on these definitions a child psychiatric illness is defined by the Department of Health and Children as

> Abnormalities of behaviour, emotions or social relationships which are sufficiently marked or prolonged to cause suffering or hardship to the child or distress or disturbance in the family or community
>
> (Department of Health, 1984: 92).

Based on the *Best Health for Children* Report (Department of Health and Children, 1999), a child is defined as being between the age of 0 and 12 years, that is approximately up to the age of puberty. Such a division does, however, provide difficulties since the provision of health services does not make a division between child and adolescent services. See chapter 6 for a discussion of adolescence and mental health.

Prevalence of mental illness in children in Ireland

One of the most serious issues in relation to discussions concerning the prevalence of mental illness in children in Ireland lies in the paucity of statistical or research material available. The UN Committee on the Rights of the Child (1998) expressed its concern about the lack of adequate epidemiological information relating to children's mental health on a national basis and highlighted the need to develop information systems to monitor trends in incidence and to identify risk factors and risk groups. However, the Annual Report of the Chief Medical Officer (Department of Health and Children, 2001c: 92) stated that 'the absence of epidemiological information relating to children's mental health on a national basis is a significant limitation in our current system'. Despite this statement the same report estimates that as many as 18 per cent of the child population under the age of sixteen years will experience significant mental health problems at some period of their development (Department of Health and Children, 2001c: 88).

The Irish College of Psychiatrists Report to the Expert Group on Mental Health (2003c), using international statistical data, estimated that overall 20 per cent of children have a mental disorder at any one time. Of these ten per cent would be mild, eight per cent would have a moderate to severe disorder and two per cent would have a disabling disorder. Boys have a higher incidence of disorders than girls but this evens out by middle to late adolescence (2003: 8). However, they argue that the potential for a higher prevalence rate exists in Ireland on the basis that the population under the age of 16 years is among the highest in Europe. The 2002 Census of the Population (CSO, 2002) showed that the percentage of the population aged 0–15 years was 22.68 per cent. This compares with 20.24 per cent in the United Kingdom and 19.04 per cent in Finland (Irish College of Psychiatrists, 2003c: 9).

Some small local studies do exist which provide limited statistical information on the prevalence of mental illness among children in Ireland. A survey carried out by the Mater Hospital Psychiatric Unit found that 20 per cent of adolescents in Ireland suffer from some form of mental health problem, depression being the most common at 6.7 per cent and anxiety disorders at 4.6 per cent (Lynch et al., 2004). Kerry Mental Health Association carried out a study of 922 children aged 12 in the county found that 6.4 per cent reported extreme levels of stress, 4.4 per cent feelings of not being able to cope, 19 per cent moderate levels of stress and 14 per cent stated that they had difficulties coping with problems in general (Hill et al., 2003). The Health Research Report on Psychiatric Services 2003 (HRB, 2004) showed that 66 children were admitted to psychiatric units, the youngest being a girl of six. The most common diagnosis for children was anxiety disorder. This compares with a total of 50 admissions of children in 2000 (Department of Health and Children, 2001b). However, these figures give no real indication of the level of mental illness among children in Ireland but are probably more indicative of the lack of services for children with psychiatric disorders.

The South Eastern Health Board and the Psychology Department at University College Dublin are currently undertaking a major research programme focusing on the mental health needs of children. The research is being undertaken in response to the Amnesty International Report (2003) which was critical of the lack of data on the mental health needs of children and the quality of information and support for children, parents and teachers in identifying mental health problems. The study will screen every child by survey in the town of Clonmel (N = approximately 5,000). Preliminary results show that more than 4,000 under 18 year olds in the town and its surrounding area have significant mental health problems which is equivalent to 17 per cent of the age group. The prevalence of mental health problems among preschool children was 12 per cent and among national schoolchildren it was 11 per cent of the age group in the study. The rate of 17 per cent is higher than that found in previous Irish epidemiological child mental health studies (Carr, 2000). However, earlier studies were with smaller samples and were confined to a narrower age range. The next stage of the study will provide information from in-depth qualitative interviews with families to determine the diagnosis and causes of the problems (Martin et al., 2005).

It is very clear that the inadequacy of statistical data on the prevalence of mental illness among the child population in Ireland militates against appropriate provision of services to meet the needs of these children. The Amnesty International Report (2003) stressed the utmost urgency of the need for the Irish government to 'regularly compile accurate data on the mental health needs of children, particularly those in vulnerable communities and in and upon leaving health board care' (Amnesty International, 2003: 38).

Children at risk of psychiatric disorder

The Irish College of Psychiatrists (2003: 9) has indicated that there are four main categories of increased risk of psychiatric disorders developing in childhood.

1   Social factors: children in urban areas are usually twice as likely to develop a disorder than those in rural areas. Children in areas of high unemployment, social disadvantage and discrimination, isolation, homelessness and family breakdown are particularly vulnerable. They are defined as at risk because they may lack child care and protection and those in the care of the health boards are also vulnerable.
2   Specific conditions: children with language and communication problems are three times more likely than the general population of children to develop mental disorders. In addition, children with developmental disorders and learning disabilities are four times more likely than the general child population to develop psychiatric disorders.
3   Stress-related conditions: children who have been physically or sexually abused are three times more likely than the general population to suffer from a psychiatric illness and children whose parents suffer from a psychiatric illness have increased rates of disorder.
4   Physical illness or disorder: children with a chronic illness have twice the general population prevalence of a disorder and where this is combined with a physical disability they are three times more likely to develop a psychiatric illness. Children with brain disorders have a five times more chance of developing such an illness as children in the general population.

Jané-Llopis (2004), in discussing prevention and promotion in mental health for children, argued that a healthy start in life enhances mental and physical health and the child's later functioning in society leading to increased social capital. Exposure to risk factors such as poor nutrition, limited access to education, poverty and social isolation, is related to poor mental health, aggressive behaviour and mental disorders which will extend through to adulthood. She emphasised the need for policy strategies that promote a healthy start in life free of poverty, free pre-school attendance from the age of three, access to high standards of education independent of income, access to effective mental health promotion components integrated in a holistic school approach, access to appropriate evidence based preventive school interventions for children and adolescents at risk of behavioural and mental disorders and community strategies for out of school and marginalised children and adolescents. In addition, she recommended services which provided training in positive, proactive parenting skills, family friendly work and welfare policies and health care policies for families at risk to increase job security and reduce income disparities and their consequences.

Current service provision

The Child and Adolescent Psychiatric Service provides mental health services for children from birth to their 16th birthday. The central principles of the service are that it is child centred, comprehensive, integrated with other health services, based as far as possible in the community and organised in sectors closest to the people being served (Irish College of Psychiatrists, 2003c: 12). Children aged between 0 and 12 years are generally seen by members of a multidisciplinary team and are almost entirely dealt with on an out-patient basis with direct and ongoing involvement of the family. The need for in-patient treatment rarely arises for children under the age of five years and irregularly for children aged between six and twelve.

The Working Group established by the Department of Health and Children in 2001 expressed the view that the most effective form of treatment of children with mental illness was through community-based services: 'the internationally best practice for the provision of child and adolescent psychiatric services is through the multi-disciplinary team' (2001b: 4). International research has also shown that community care is more effective than in-patient care (Pilgrim and Rogers, 1999; Jacob and Greene, 1998). Most of the assessment, treatment and care of children with mental health needs in Ireland is in fact provided in the community by community-based teams. At the pre-school level, assessment and treatment programmes are run by a clinic nurse and a childcare worker. The community multidisciplinary teams also run a number of groups such on social skills, anxiety management or parenting. Assessment and treatment of school-going children usually involves clinic work with single or multi-disciplinary approaches using individual and family work provided through a variety of skills and treatment options such as psychotherapy, pharmacotherapy, family therapy, cognitive behavioural therapy and activity-based therapies such as play, art, music and drama therapy (Irish College of Psychiatrists, 2003c: 16). However, the number of teams falls far short of the number estimated to meet the needs of these children. At the present time there are 35 multidisciplinary community teams despite the recommendation from the *First Report from the Working Group on Child and Adolescent Psychiatric Service* (Department of Health and Children, 2001a), which recommended a complement of 120 which would be equivalent to one team per 100,000 population.

While the above represents the ideal situation, the actual provision of services has been found to be inadequate in relation to demand. The Irish College of Psychiatrists points out that the child psychiatric services have traditionally provided out-patient services only, often with limited resources and with restricted access to in-patient beds or day hospital facilities. At the present time in-patient services are severely under resourced to meet demand. The *First Report from the Working Group on Child and Adolescent Psychiatric*

Services (Department of Health and Children, 2001a) recommended the provision of 144 in-patient beds and the development of seven new child and adolescent psychiatric units. This compares with the actual provision of 20 in-patient beds for the entire country. In comparison, Finland with a population of 5.2 million has 290 in-patient beds (Irish College of Psychiatrists, 2003c: 18).

In May 2004 Our Lady's Hospital for Sick Children in Dublin requested the Eastern Regional Health Authority to consider the possibility of sending children with acute mental health problems requiring in-patient treatment out of the jurisdiction in order to meet their needs. As one consultant child psychiatrist commented:

> In Dublin there are no emergency child psychiatric beds available and this has led to many of these children being detained in the hospital for extended periods of time inappropriately and often without the correct legal framework to do so (*Irish Times Health Supplement*, 20 May 2004).

A similar deficit exists in human resources. For example, the number of consultant child psychiatrists expressed as a ratio of the population aged 0–15 years is 1:18,200 (total of 49 consultants) compared to 1: 6,000 in Finland, 1: 7,000 in Sweden and 1: 7,500 in France.

The Irish College of Psychiatrists (2003c: 34–5) has highlighted the gaps in the service provision as follows:

• Shortage of consultant child psychiatrists
• Existing teams serving excessive number of population
• Teams below the complement recommended by the *First Report from the Working Group on Child and Adolescent Psychiatric Services* (Department of Health and Children, 2001a)
• Shortage of trained staff in key disciplines e.g. psychologists, social workers and occupational and speech therapists
• Demand exceeding resources due to deficiencies in primary care services
• Inadequate accommodation for some teams
• Gaps and under-resourcing of in-patient services
• Incomplete liaison teams in major paediatric hospitals
• Lack of consultant psychiatric sessions in paediatric units
• No infant psychiatric service

Specific disorders in children

The services for children with specific disorders have been highlighted within government reports, reports from the Irish College of Psychiatrists and from special interest parent support groups.

1 Attention Deficit Disorder (ADHD)

The Irish College of Psychiatrists (2003c: 26) has estimated that between one and five per cent of school age children suffer from ADHD. This is equivalent to approximately 18,000 children. Currently only a small proportion of these children are referred to specialist child and adolescent psychiatric services. It is estimated that with increasing recognition of this condition in the community the number of children referred for assessment will have serious resource implications. The *First Report of the Working Group on Child and Adolescent Psychiatric Services* (Department of Health and Children, 2001a) concluded that the enhancement and expansion of child and adolescent services through-out the country would represent the best forward plan for meeting the needs of children with ADHD. However, it is clear that the effective working of such teams can be hampered by shortages in supporting professions such as educational psychologists and specialist teaching posts. Such deficits lead to difficulties in the development of a school-based treatment service for children with ADHD.

2 Autistic Spectrum Disorder (ASD)

The number of cases of ASD has shown significant increase worldwide with an estimated prevalence of 60 in every 10,000 children. In Ireland the Irish College of Psychiatrists (2003c: 27) estimate that there are 5,330 children with this disorder ranging from those with severe difficulties to those with lesser problems affecting understanding and impaired social functioning. It is also estimated that approximately half of them also have some level of intellectual disability.

Early assessment and diagnosis have been linked with maximising the outcome for the children with ASD and in the provision of support for the families and siblings. However, specialist autism services have developed in an uneven manner and community teams do not have the resources to carry out early assessments and treatment.

The *Report on Services for Persons with Autism* (Department of Health, 1994a) specified that services should

- Be specific to the triad of impairments characterising autism
- Have an approach that is tailored to individual needs
- Involve parents as partners
- Be localised

A study by Doherty et al. (2003: 148–64) of 85 individuals with autism and their families involved interviewing the primary caregiver of each of the participants and their key workers. The study found that over one third of the key workers had received no training in autism and older clients compared with younger clients were significantly less likely to have an individual educational plan in place. Overall service satisfaction was good but caregivers wanted more parental involvement in service provision and to have an assurance of ongoing care for the individual with autism. The study's findings suggested a need for more partnership between parents and staff in the care and education of individuals with autism together with more respite and support for the caregivers.

3 Asperger's Syndrome

Asperger's syndrome (Gillberg, 1991) includes six criteria for its diagnosis: social impairments, narrow interests, repetitive routines, speech and language peculiarities, non-verbal communication problems and motor clumsiness. The American Psychiatric Association (1994) based their diagnostic criteria on impairment in social interaction and the presence of stereotypic or repetitive behaviours. Diagnosis must be based on a clinically significant level of impairment and occur before the age of three (Fitzgerald and Corvin, 2003: 82).

Fitzgerald and Corvin (2003: 82–96) examine the difficulties in diagnosing Asperger's syndrome emphasising the possibility of misdiagnosing it in relation to a variety of similar but contrasting conditions. They argue that diagnostic confusion arises because many disorders such as ADHD, autism, dyslogia, Rett's disorder and schizoid personality disorders present with similar symptoms. Such confusion then places increased burdens on individuals and families because they 'seek unhelpful therapies or join the wrong support groups' (Fitzgerald and Corvin, 2003: 90). They emphasise the need for early and correct diagnosis using a multidisciplinary team approach rather than a solely neurological, speech and language or educational point of view. However, to undertake early diagnosis and treatment from a multidisciplinary approach obviously requires adequate resources and, as for other major child psychiatric disorders, these services are currently inadequate.

The sudden rise in the number of young children who have been diagnosed with an attention deficit disorder has placed enormous demands on both the health and educational services. The inability of the state to respond effectively to the needs of these children and their families has led to numerous High Court actions by parents and to the publication of reports such as the *Report of the Task Force on Autism* (Department of Education, 2001), the *Review of Services for Persons with Autistic Spectrum Disorders* (Eastern Regional Health Authority, 2002b) and the *Review of the Needs and Services for Children and Young People with Asperger's in the Area Health Boards of the Eastern Region* (South Western Area Health Board, 2001). The Psychological Society of Ireland in their submission to the Expert Group on Mental Health Services stresses the urgency of implementing the recommendations of these various report (Psychological Society of Ireland, 2003c). In particular, they consider there is a need for considerable expansion of early diagnostic and assessment services, early intervention services coupled with clinical supports such as parent counselling and training, occupational therapy, speech and language therapy, behavioural supports, respite care, home support services and residential services. They consider that the psychological/psychiatric services are in need of expansion and a co-ordinated approach from health and education in the delivery of services is required.

It is clear that services for those children with autistic spectrum disorders vary enormously across the state with many areas having no health support services. Where services exist they are insufficiently resourced to cope with the demands.

Child mental health policy

The World Health Organisation's *Mental Health Policy Project* (WHO, 2001) stated that

> there is a virtual worldwide absence of an identifiable national child and adolescent mental health policy . . . a comprehensive national child and adolescent mental health policy can facilitate the ability to gather more precise epidemiological data essential for treatment and prevention program development tailored to country needs. Without policy guidance for child and adolescent mental health there is a very real danger that fragmented ineffective systems of care will emerge or be sustained. In this case, competing constituencies and agencies inevitably provide a less than adequate product for a cost that exceeds expectations

The report emphasised that a good collaborative planning and policy development process driven by a formal national policy can result in cost efficiencies and provide a continuum of care that benefits the recipient, child, adolescent, family and community.

It is very clear from an examination of successive Irish documents published in the area of health and children that there is no overall vision or policy in relation to the mental health needs of children, either as to current needs or in prevention. The Irish Psychiatric Association (2003) argued that the absence of an up-to-date national mental health strategy is one of the main causes of current inequities in the distribution or resources within the mental health field. They state that the resources have been concentrated not in areas of greatest need but in areas of greatest affluence. This has been echoed by the Irish College of Psychiatrists (2003c: 1) on the need to develop a new national mental health policy immediately.

The mental health strategy document *The Psychiatric Services: Planning for the Future* (Department of Health, 1984) remains the framework for a national policy on mental health concentrating as it does on the need for community care provision for both adults and children and an orientation towards a holistic approach through multidisciplinary co-operation within the health, social and educational services.

In 1999 the report *Best Health for Children: Developing a Partnership with Families* (Department of Health and Children, 1999) sought to develop a strategy that would place families and children at the centre of service provision. It argued that emotional and psychological health needs of children have received insufficient attention in the overall health promotion of children and families. The report recommended the development of improved detection and treatment services. In terms of the latter they proposed that there should be appropriately sited in-patient facilities staffed with specialist services. This report also identified the wider causal and risk factors for child mental health as socio-economic disadvantage, family discord, families with existing psychiatric illness and learning difficulties. The identification of these factors highlights the need for a broadly based mental health policy aimed at preventive measures linked with the *National Anti-Poverty Strategy* (Government of Ireland, 1997) and the *National Children's Strategy* (Department of Health and Children, 2000a)

The *National Children's Strategy* (Department of Health and Children, 2000) specifically mentions mental health services for children as in need of reform as it states that services to meet the mental health and emotional needs of children continue to need expansion (2000: 7). The *National Children's Strategy* also emphasises the need to develop community services for children and the development of health promotion in line with best international practice. In addition it recommends the development of a health strategy to guide mental health services for children and adolescents. (2000: 92)

The emphasis on health promotion is also contained within the *Annual Report of the Chief Medical Officer of Health* (Department of Health and Children, 2001c). This report highlights the need for policies to target the links between mental illness and social factors and to develop programmes which emphasise mental and emotional health, self esteem, personal relationships and coping capacities.

The national health strategy *Quality and Fairness: A Health System for You* (Department of Health and Children, 2001b) contains a small section on mental health and within that section children are mentioned only briefly and few of the over 100 recommendations proposed in relation to goals, objectives, actions and targets refer explicitly to mental health measures. However, it did recommend updating *The Psychiatric Services: Planning for the Future* (Department of Health, 1984) to produce a new national mental health strategy. No such measure has yet been undertaken. *Quality and Fairness: A Health System For You – Action Plan Progress Report 2003* (Department of Health and Children,

2003b) commented that the *Working Group on Child and Adolescent Psychiatry* (March 2001) had recommended that seven child and adolescent in-patient psychiatric units for children ranging from six to 16 years should be developed throughout the country and by 2003 project teams had been established in respect of four of the proposed units.

In the light of the fact that the precipitating factors in child mental health problems are often rooted in the family situation, there has been a move to invest in family support projects as a preventative measure. Since 2002 ongoing funding in excess of €12 million has been provided for support services including the Springboard Family Support Projects. Funding to establish four Springboard Projects in RAPID/priority areas was provided in 2002 and a fifth project in 2003 giving a total of 22 projects throughout the country. The Best Health for Children Programme provides for a new core surveillance programme for all children aged 0–12 years with pre-school development examinations as well as the school health service.

The *First Report of the Inspector of Mental Health Services* (Inspector of Mental Health Services, 2004) stated that a priority of the Inspectorate for 2004 was to carry out an audit of mental health service provision for children and adolescents and those with intellectual disability. The Inspector considered that the child mental health services were underdeveloped, and recommended that the child and adolescent mental health services require one specialist team for each 100,000 population with the number of consultants and therapists depending on local factors such as family structure and deprivation levels. The report also recommended that child and adolescent mental health services be available on a 24-hour, seven-day basis and in a position to respond to emergency referrals.

Conclusions

In Ireland, development of a strategy and policies for the delivery of services for children with mental health problems has been slow and integrated within general health strategies rather than as specialist provision. It has also been an area which has been under-resourced within the totality of health services. The emphasis on treatment of children presenting with mental health problems rather than the development of a preventive approach has also been evident. However, Ireland is not alone. The World Health Organisation's *Mental Health Policy Project* pointed out that there is a virtual worldwide absence of an identifiable national child and adolescent mental health policy (WHO, 2001c). In addition, the WHO/EU Pre-Conference on Child and Adolescent Mental Health held in Luxembourg September 2004 highlighted the fact that policies and services for children with mental health problems are in general underdeveloped and under resourced across a wide range of countries.

In order to achieve best practice in child mental health a number of current gaps in the services need to be addressed. These include gaps in multi-disciplinary teams, specialist child services particularly for children with ASD and ADHD, in-patient services, day hospital programmes, programmes for children with eating disorders and evaluation audits and research. (Irish College of Psychiatrists, 2003c)

It is very clear that the development of any strategy for the delivery of mental health services for children must be evidence based. The prevalence of childhood behavioural disorders and psychiatric disorders needs to be quantified by national research to ensure that there is a sound basis on which to develop policies and strategies to meet the needs of this group and their families. A national mental health policy aimed specifically at children should be developed. Such a policy could then provide a set of guidelines to inform services. Rapid social change with a pressure to succeed, as well as commercial and media influences are shaping the mental health of children and their families in a more affluent society in which increasing numbers of families are breaking down adding to stress levels for children.

One further issue that needs to be addressed is the matter of children's rights. Under the UN Convention on the Rights of the Child (1989) Article 24.1 states that

> States Parties recognise the right of the child to the enjoyment of the highest attainable standard of health and to facilities for the treatment of illness and rehabilitation of health. States Parties shall strive to ensure that no child is deprived of his or her right of access to such health care services.

In addition, thirty of the Convention's articles have some direct or indirect relationship to the impact of violence and trauma on children and adolescents. Garrison (2004: 228) argues that several of these articles can be applied in assuring the protection of basic rights of children and adolescents who experience emotional and behavioural disorders. The theme of the World Federation for Mental Health's 2003 World Mental Health Day was on advocating a global mental health education campaign. It emphasised the need for increased understanding and attention to the mental and emotional health needs of children and young people. It promoted increased advocacy to encourage national governments to develop and implement child mental health policies that would foster improved funding, services and accountability within national mental health programmes servicing this group. The campaign also emphasised the need for increased attention to be paid to children with mental health problems and to do so from a children's rights perspective.

Without policy guidance on child mental health within countries, the World Health Organisation considers that there is a very real danger that fragmented, ineffective systems of care will emerge or be sustained. In this case competing constituencies and agencies inevitably provide a less than adequate product for a cost that exceeds expectations (WHO, 2001b). The Mental Health Project on child and adolescent mental health concluded that,

> Good collaborative planning and policy development process driven by a formal national policy can result in cost efficiencies and provide a continuum of care that benefits the recipient ... child, adolescent, family and community (WHO, 2001c)

In order to assist in the development of child mental health strategies the WHO Mental Health Policy and Service Guidance Package (WHO, 2005a) has been developed to assist policy makers and planners to develop a policy and comprehensive strategy for improving the mental health of children, to use existing resources to achieve the greatest possible benefits, provide effective services to those children in need and assist the reintegration of persons with mental disorders into all aspects of community life. The Guidance Package identifies *inter alia* five guiding principles for a comprehensive policy for child mental health planning and development. These principles are financing, legislation and human rights, advocacy, quality improvement, organisation of services and planning and budgeting. (WHO, 2005a: xi) They argue that funding sources need to recognise the long-term commitment to allow for positive outcomes and funding needs to be aimed at developing a continuum of care. Child mental health policy is most effective when it encompasses a framework that relates child development and an understanding of the rights of the child. Child mental health advocacy by parents, professionals and the young people themselves is an important element of policy development by facilitating an understanding of the issues and to convey to the public at large the rationale for the implementation and financing of services for this group of children. The organisation and quality improvement aspect of any services must be grounded in evidence-based best practice. The planning and budgeting for service delivery require adequate information on the local and national needs for services and the relative allocation of funds across other health sectors and sectors of the general national economy.

Taking a holistic approach to the development of a mental health policy for children should be the underlying principle. Such a view recognises and builds on the strengths and capacities of families. Within this holistic approach children and families at particular risk should be targeted. These might include children whose parents suffer from mental illness or enduring physical illness, from high levels of social deprivation and poverty who have experienced particularly stressful life events or are suffering from post traumatic stress. Thus policies should be aimed at addressing the social risk factors known to underlie mental health problems. These include inequality, stigma, marginalisation, social exclusion and poverty. By developing strong and supportive mental well being infrastructures the possibility arises for a move to a preventive approach rather than a reactive one.

It is clear that what is required is an emphasis on mental health promotion through school-based programmes and pre-school parenting programmes. Improving the psychosocial quality of life of children and raising public awareness about children's needs are important pillars of child mental health protection and need to be the starting point for the development of a strategy for child mental health.

Chapter 6

Adolescence and mental health

Suzanne Quin
Victoria Richardson

Introduction

This chapter will focus on adolescence as a life stage that poses particular challenges and risks for mental health associated with transition to adulthood. Relative to other life stages, adolescence in Ireland as in other westernised societies is characterised by low morbidity and mortality (CSO, 2002). Nevertheless, mental health disorders in adolescence do occur and can be divided into two categories. First of all, there are those that are diagnosed in childhood and continue on into adolescence. The second group is disorders that are more likely to develop during the adolescent phase. These include depressive disorders and eating disorders, the latter in particular associated with adolescent girls.

A particular feature of adolescence is engagement in risk behaviours. The term 'risk behaviours' covers a wide range of activities including alcohol and drug abuse, speeding, participating in hazardous sports as well as having potentially harmful eating patterns. Taken together, risk behaviours pose a significant threat to the health and well being of many adolescents. Some of the risk factors more than others tend to be gender specific. In the context of overall mental health policy and service provision for adolescents, specific attention will be given to one type of risk behaviour – eating disorders. These disorders are important because they are complex in terms of aetiology and interventions, predominantly affect females and have potentially very harmful consequences for the increasing numbers of those affected.

Adolescence as a life stage

The period of adolescence is of vital developmental importance. The term adolescent refers to any young person between the ages of 12 to 18 (National Conjoint Child Health Committee, 2000). The extent to which young people can effectively adjust to adult life depends largely on their personal strengths, family support and circumstances, personal relationships, training and environmental factors and of course the state of their mental health. Common presentations of mental health problems in adolescence encompass emotional upset, deviant behaviour, poor school performance or attendance, eating disorders, alcohol and drug abuse. Assessment of mental health presents a number of challenges to mental health professionals. A developmental perspective is crucial in assessing and treating adolescents since both level of functioning and presenting disorders must be viewed in the context of developmental norms. Although adolescence is a time of immense change both physically and emotionally, 'no psychiatric diagnoses are specific to adolescence: most adult and child psychiatric disorders are seen, often modified by the patient's developmental stage' (Katona and Robertson, 2000: 52)

A particular feature of modernity is the increasing time of dependency between childhood and adulthood. Adolescents are exposed to a myriad of influences: family, peer, educational as well as the media in its many forms. In western society, adolescence as a life stage is characterised by peer attachment, seeking independence from the family while simultaneously being economically and practically dependent, adjusting to physiological change as well as developing a sense of identity and self-worth. The complexity of tasks can pose significant challenges for adolescents. Magnusson (WHO, 2004) comments that 'it is of great concern that modern life appears to put so much pressure on young people that their mental health is affected'. In turn, the presence of a mental health disorder can affect the adolescent's ability to successfully accomplish these tasks. The National Conjoint Child Health Committee (2000: 3) stated that 'mental health for adolescents can be influenced, positively or negatively, by the developmental tasks involved in this transitional period of life. It is a time when experimental behaviour is a core part of negotiating these tasks'.

Risk behaviours are often regarded as one of the hallmarks of adolescence. That this may be a facet of modern, westernised societies, is indicated by Cole and Cole (1996: 646), who cite cross-cultural evidence that high levels of risk taking are not a universal feature of adolescence. As Kelley et al. (2004) point out, risk taking and novelty seeking have adaptive benefits in the development of independence and survival but they also leave the adolescent vulnerable to harm. Given that adolescence can be a time of high risk in terms of lifestyle with potential long-term consequences, it is not surprising that health policy views adolescents as important targets for health promotion.

One target set out in the *Health Promotion Strategy 2001–2005* (Department of Health and Children, 2001b) is to encourage healthy eating patterns among children and adolescents. There is concern both about overeating resulting in obesity as well as excessive dieting with its associated health risks of developing into an eating disorder. The *Irish Health Behaviour in School-Aged Children* study (Friel et al., 1999) found that 25 per cent of a large-scale sample of almost 8,500 9–17 year olds thought that they should be on a diet.

Adolescent mental health

Adolescence is a time of constant change coupled with a desire for increased independence and reluctance to share difficulties with adult figures. The Irish College of Psychiatrists (2002) has recognised that it is a period of increased vulnerability to mental health difficulties and they have highlighted the increased incidence and prevalence. In the past 50 years, Western Europe has seen a rise in identified psychological disorders among children and adolescents, including eating disorders, drug and alcohol misuse, criminal behaviour, self-harm and attempted suicide (Rutter and Smith, 1995). However, with the increase in prevalence, policy and services have been slow to respond to the constant increase in need arising from this group. In 1977 the WHO proposed the need for every country to establish a national plan for child mental health. Almost thirty years on, Shatkin and Belfer (2004) undertook a study which aimed to establish the number of countries worldwide that possessed a national mental healthy policy for children and adolescents. Their findings concluded that no one country has a comprehensive mental health policy for children and adolescents.

Epidemiological studies of mental health disorders in adolescence show that about 15 per cent of the adolescent population in western society have a mental disorder. One quarter of these will have significant functional impairment (National Conjoint Child Health Committee, 2001). Applying these figures to the Irish population, it can be estimated that approximately 87,000 adolescents in Ireland suffer from a mental disorder of some kind (CSO, 2002). By late adolescence girls have a significantly higher rate of mental disorders than boys. However, such gender differences may be more related to differences in presentation and treatment of behaviour problems. Nevertheless, based on known incidence, the fact that adolescent females have a much higher propensity to eating disorders than adolescent males, is an important factor in overall gender differences in mental disorders in adolescence. In terms of response to mental health problems, it is estimated that only a small fraction of adolescents with mental health problems are in contact with helping agencies (National Conjoint Child Health Committee, 2001).

Prevalence of eating disorders

While young children can be at risk, eating disorders usually emerge during adolescence (Polivy et al., 2003: 523). Polivy et al. (2003: 537) point out that for decades researchers assumed that eating disorders were a feature of privileged,

Caucasian populations. However, it has now been demonstrated that eating disorders are a global phenomenon found across different ethnic and racial populations and socio-economic groups while prevalence rates are found to be higher among Caucasian and industrialised nations. Fombonne (1995: 638), reviewing studies of prevalence rates, commented that the results showed a clear difference between the rates of prevalence found in Asian countries in contrast to those of Europe, North America, Australia and New Zealand. Jones et al. (2001) cite research evidence to indicate that the prevalence of such disorders is rising while the age of onset is falling. In their own study of over 1,700 girls aged between 12 and 18 and attending schools in a number of different locations in Ontario, Canada, the self-reporting scales found distortions in eating attitudes and behaviours in over one quarter of respondents which increased with age. In another large-scale study of over 2,000 young people in Denmark, Waaddegaard and Peterson (2002) found that weight-loss desire and behaviours increased with age and were more related to perceptions of being overweight than actual obesity.

The Hautala Report to the European Commission (Hautala, 1999) focused on women's health and referred to eating disorders as a growing health problem which could have serious consequences for those affected, as an immediate and a long-term risk to life and health. Although not within the age range under consideration in this chapter, it is important to note that the report quoted figures of 1 in 25 women under 35 years suffering from an eating disorder. The fact that females were significantly more affected than males indicates the important role of the culture of slenderness in modern western society (Madrid et al., 2001). Fombonne (1995: 659) suggests that an important factor to consider is that 'running counter to changes in body ideal, the average weight of young women has tended to increase regularly'. This is on account of the trends across recent generations of taller and bigger build because of changes in nutrition and improvements in the general health of the population.

Eating disorders are broken down into two broad categories, both of which involve prioritising weight control (Bennett, 2003: 281). Anorexia nervosa is characterised by excessive dieting leading to weight loss accompanied by an excessive fear of weight gain. Bulimia nervosa is characterised by a cycle of dieting, binge eating and compensatory behaviours such as vomiting, use of diuretics and /or laxatives, and excessive exercise. According to Mitchell and Carr (2000: 236), eating disorders occur in about three to four per cent of the adolescent female population. This is broken down into approximately one per cent suffering from anorexia nervosa and between one and three per cent having bulimia nervosa. These authors state that adolescents with eating disorders may also engage in 'a variety of self-destructive behaviours including self-injurious behaviour, suicide attempts and drug abuse' (2000: 235–6).

Causation

There are two basic models for understanding the aetiology of eating disorders. The first (associated with the so called medical model) considers eating disorders to be a form of psychiatric illness that may exist alone or may co-exist with another mental illness, especially depression. In examining the relationship between certain psychiatric conditions and eating disorders, Zaider et al.'s (2002) research findings indicated that adolescents with chronic depressive symptoms 'may be at markedly elevated risk for the onset of BN (bulimia nervosa) or BED (binge eating disorder)'. This, they state, supports a growing body of evidence that depression can play an important role in the development of eating disorders (2002: 326).

The second model is based on a continuity hypothesis. This views eating disorders as one end of a continuum concerning problem eating that is to be found in a significant number of adolescents, particularly females, in westernised societies. In this model, the focus is on trying to identify the important variables that determine how some adolescents move from problem eating to an eating disorder that is dangerous to their life and well being. A study by Kansi et al. (2003) investigated the variation of eating problems in a representative sample of over 5,000 adolescent girls in Norway. The researchers found 'initial support for the continuity hypothesis regarding eating problems characterised by bulimic tendencies and dieting [and] . . . no clear support regarding restrictive eating problems' (2003: 333). They identified low self-esteem as an important factor in the likelihood of developing an eating problem.

Seeking to understand why and who will develop an eating disorder in adolescence has led to many potential causal factors being identified. Polivy et al. (2003) divide these into the following broad categories:

1   Individual – biological factors including genetic influences as well as neurotransmitters and hormonal influences
2   Psychological – pubertal issues such as changes in body shape and increase in body fat for pubescent girls, body image and associated dieting and involvement in activities emphasising weight/shape
3   Emotional – personality traits such as perfectionism and negative self-evaluation
4   Family – such as parental influences, family interaction patterns and issues relating to autonomy, self-control and identity
5   Socio-cultural – including media influences, gender role expectations as well as race, ethnicity and social class

The role of the media

Much attention has been focused on the role of the media on the lifestyle and self-image of adolescents in contemporary society. Writing about the United

States yet of no less relevance to here, Santrock (2002: 348) comments that 'today's adolescents face demands and expectation, as well as risks and temptations, that appear to be more numerous and complex than those faced by adolescents only a generation ago'. This, Santrock (2002: 348–9) attributes to adolescents being exposed to a complex menu of lifestyle options through the media. The globalisation of lifestyle encouraged by the mass media and the web means that adolescents are aware of and identify with life stage commonalities than transcend geographical and socio-economic divisions.

The role of the media in the causation of eating disorders cannot be definitively proven. Nevertheless, it is evident that the media play a role in the development of self-image and in presenting role models of body image. The current preoccupation with the presentation of thin pre-pubertal, waiflike appearance in the fashion and film industries hardly provides realistic and healthy body-image role models for adolescent girls. 'Women and girls in postmodern societies are bombarded with messages from the media, parents and peers that the ideal body is one that is almost impossibly thin' (Klaczynski et al., 2004: 308).

In examining trends in reported incidence in anorexia nervosa over decades in different locations, Fombonne (1995: 621–6) refers to the Rochester Study in America, which examined trends over a period of 50 years from 1935 to 1985. It found clear variations over time, leading the researchers to speculate that 'the number of more severe cases may have remained steady, whereas the fluctuations may have been in the number of less severe cases'. They further suggested that the fluctuations identified might have been in response to changes in women's fashion, which emphasised thinness in the 1920s, then more curvaceous forms after the Second World War, then thinness again in the 1960s. Since the 1960s, 'images of femininity and female attractiveness have shifted . . . to a slimmer, less "hour glass" shape' (Bennett, 2003: 286). Polivy et al. (2003: 536) comment that 'the media portrayals of body shapes impossible for most girls to attain appear to be at the least a contributing factor to body dissatisfaction, disordered eating behaviours, and outright eating disorders in susceptible adolescent girls'.

This point is further emphasised by Cole and Cole (1996: 636–7) that

> the message to girls in our [US] society comes across as loud and clear: being beautiful means being thin. Images of tall, lithe models with boyish figures smile at us from the covers of the fashion magazines. Thin, young actresses are the objects of desire in popular movies . . . It is no wonder then, that most adolescent girls in our society are afraid of being fat.

A study by Vincent and McCabe of over 600 adolescents in Melbourne, Australia led the researchers to comment that 'girls are continually exposed to a subculture that values and promotes the slender ideal, where such issues are reinforced via discussions amongst parents and peers' (2000: 218).

Development of policy for adolescents with eating disorders

Eating disorders in adolescence are clearly relevant to mental health policy and service development. The importance of preventative as well as curative interventions is evident. Newman and Newman (2003) comment that while 'the origins of eating disorders are not fully understood' many writers on the topic 'implicate the cultural infatuation with thinness as a stimulus of this condition'. Hence, they refer to the value of creating a social climate that promotes 'a more positive acceptance of people of various body types and shapes, with less focus on thinness' (Newman and Newman, 2003: 303–4). The role of the media is important creating more positive attitudes. As well as the images and messages they portray, it is important to understand how the media are used in adolescents' daily lives, as well as the forces determining how the media are created and deployed (Mastronardi, 2003).

The findings of Wertheim et al.'s (2001: 79) study of adolescent girls in Australia suggest that by the time of mid adolescence, eating behaviours become relatively stable and those with problem eating patterns that have developed by that time are likely to continue. They suggest that the appropriate timing for intervention programmes may be pre/early adolescence, which is supported by the findings of Hargreaves and Tiggermann (2003), who found that viewing television commercials that included idealised female thin images increased body dissatisfaction in girls as young as 13 years of age. How to recognise those who are potentially more likely to develop an eating disorder as early as possible is clearly a priority. Pratt et al. (2003) highlight the need for further research on the protective as well as the risk factors that could help to predict those vulnerable to the development of an eating disorder.

Mental health policy and services for adolescents in Ireland

The Child Care Act 1991 defines a child as anyone under the age of 18, although an anomaly exists between this and the provision of mental health services in Ireland. Mental health services for the Irish population are divided into Child and Adolescent Services which provide a service up to age 16 and Adult Psychiatric Services which are are responsible for those aged 18 and over. This creates a two-year gap at a significant transient stage of life between adolescence and embarking on adult life. The implementation of the Mental Health Act 2001 raised the age to bring it in line with the provisions set out under the Child Care Act 1991. This does not, however, alter the implications and present dearth in the provision of services to adolescents with mental health difficulties.

Recent Irish statistics for the year 2003 reveal that there were 66 admissions to children's centres for the treatment of mental health difficulties. Fifty-five per cent of all admissions were female. It is recorded that almost one quarter (23 per cent) of all admissions were aged 16, one fifth (21 per cent) were aged 14 with a further 18 per cent aged 15 (Daly et al., 2004: 115). The statistics highlight the need to make service provision for the adolescent population a priority.

The current child and adolescent services are mainly provided in out-patient settings. There are three in-patient units in the country for children and adolescents with mental health problems. These are located only in Dublin and Galway where service provision and catchment area are generally reserved for their own regions. There are no in-patient settings available for individuals over the age of 16 and only one day hospital currently provides a service to this age group. A census carried out on the profile of patients on one particular night in an adult psychiatric in-patient facility in 2001 revealed that there were 88 people aged between 16 and 19 receiving care (Irish College of Psychiatrists, 2003a: 1). The Working Group on Child and Adolescent Psychiatric Services stressed that the treatment of adolescents within adult mental health services is inappropriate because of the lack of resources for dealing with them (Department of Health and Children, 2003c). The Working Group found that it was difficult to establish how many adolescents were receiving psychiatric input from an adult service, as there was a lack of information relating to referrals and non-attendance at out-patient clinics.

The Working Group has identified that psychiatric services for adolescents require the involvement of a multidisciplinary team headed by a consultant Child and Adolescent Psychiatrist and members of staff with an expertise and knowledge of adolescents. The teams should comprise Senior Registrar, Registrar, Psychologist, Social Worker, Psychiatric Nurses, Occupational Therapist, Speech and Language Therapist and a Child Care Worker. The service on offer should include a day hospital service encompassing skills training and personal development through group therapy offering a supportive and educational approach. Assertive outreach programmes are recommended as a method of providing nursing and supportive services based in the home and school. In-patient services are to be made available with a view to providing acute, same-day admissions. The Working Group recognised that it is important to keep the number of in-patient admissions for this age group low and suggested a liaison with the general hospitals and the development of a rehabilitative aspect to the adolescent service providing community-based services as a 'step-down' service in aiding the recovery process. The Working Group also highlighted the need for a flexible approach to service provision and the importance of a commitment to providing continuous care from adolescence through to adulthood.

The World Health Organisation defines health as 'a state of complete physical, mental and social well-being' (WHO, 2004b: 17). Young people are educated on the importance of sustaining their physical well-being, yet the same emphasis is lacking with respect to their mental health. Mental Health Ireland and 'Aware' have therefore looked at methods of educating adolescents about mental health. 'Aware' have a programme called 'Beat the Blues', an awareness programme aimed at senior classes to provide greater understanding of depression and to encourage adolescents to recognise and speak about emotional problems.

Mental Health Ireland has created a programme called 'Mental Health Matters', to be integrated into the social and health component and transition-year programmes in schools. This resource pack is aimed at 14–18 year olds to:

- Address the issue of mental health in a realistic, relevant and age-appropriate manner
- Present mental health as a distinct concept integral to daily lives, the maintenance of which is vital to physical health
- Provide resource material which, in its methodology and content, is infor-mative for any school that intends to introduce a module on mental health into Transition Year
- Challenge young people's attitudes and misconceptions regarding mental illness
- Look critically at society's attitude to mental illness and the factors which influence such attitudes
- Make young people aware of the mental health services and facilities available should they, a member of their family, or a friend need to make use of them (Mental Health Ireland, 2001)

Challenges for the future

It has been suggested that mental health problems in young people are a good predictor of problems in adulthood (Achenbach et al., 1995). This would suggest that introduction to supportive and educational strategies in mental health is of paramount importance during adolescence. Outside the family, school is one of the primary socialising and learning environments.

In its report on Ireland, the UN Committee on the Rights of the Child (United Nations Committee, 1998) noted the lack of adequate programmes and services addressing the mental health of children and families. The importance of developing mental health services in Ireland is recognised in the current Health Strategy (Department of Health and Children, 2001b: 164). It acknowledges the special needs of those with eating disorders in the development of mental health services overall. An Expert Group (Department of Health and Children, 2003c) has been established to develop a framework for a national mental health policy.

The Amnesty International Report (2003) on children's mental health in Ireland recommended that service development for children and adolescents become a priority. It regarded current provision of mental health services for this group as inadequate with only a fraction of those with mental health problems receiving the necessary services. This is supported by data from the Irish College of Psychiatrists (2004: 7) indicating that Child and Adolescent Psychiatry has waiting lists of a year or more. One of its key recommendations concerns the funding and development of services for adolescents (2004: 9).

Mental Health Ireland, in promoting positive mental health amongst adolescents, has also developed a National Speaking Project to raise 'awareness among young people of the importance of positive mental health and of the causes and effects of mental illness' (Mental Health Ireland, 2001). They have also developed an Internet-based magazine for teenagers dealing with mental health issues. This is a valuable method of using a popular means of communication to which young people are familiar and have easy access for addressing aspects of mental health.

It has been suggested that young people do not necessarily recognise symptoms of ill health and are not familiar with service provision and so they are slower than others in accessing existing services. Consequently, the National Cojoint Committee (2004: 17) recommended that the provision of facilities be orientated towards the needs and experiences of this age group. Education and service provision are thus intrinsically linked and need to be addressed in relation to each other and not separately.

Incorporating adolescents' voices in service planning and delivery

The World Health Organisation, in considering the components of a balanced care mental health service, emphasises the importance of primary care. Thus it recommends that 'primary care training to recognise and treat mental disorders should be given high priority, so that such skills form part of primary care givers' core expertise' (WHO, 2000b: 1). It also views adolescence along with childhood as needing to be prioritised in the development of mental health services.

The National Conjoint Child Health Committee (2000) has pointed out that the health of young people is important for their current situation and is vital for the health of the future population, as 'it is in adolescence that the foundations of future health are laid' (2000: 3.3). It suggests that the provision of [health care] facilities should take cognisance of the needs and experiences of adolescents by involving them in the planning, delivery and evaluation of services so that 'their ideas in relation to health-related problems become a key resource for health action' (2000: 3.1).

Conclusion

Adolescence is a time of challenge and vulnerability, most particularly for those with mental health problems. Current services are insufficient to offer the range and level of intervention required to address their needs. There is scope for further development of curative and preventative services. Ensuring that the 'adolescent voice' is heard in both policy planning and service delivery is vital so that what is on offer is appropriate and acceptable. We have focused on one aspect of adolescent mental health in particular – eating disorders – as these pose a particular threat to a significant proportion of adolescent girls. Intervention is needed at a number of levels to address this important health issue. At curative level, the quantity and range of interventions on offer need expansion; at preventative level programmes are needed to highlight the pressures and risks associated with inappropriate eating and dieting. The question of how the ideal body type is selected and portrayed in society should be tackled. Involvement by adolescents in addressing this problem at each level is a vital component of finding more effective ways of dealing with this important issue.

Chapter 7

Mental health and suicide

Mary Allen

Introduction

Comprehensive mental health policy is an important element in supporting people to deal with the pressures of modern living. A symptom of the effects of extreme pressures has been the alarming increase in Irish suicide rates. However, unlike many other issues relating to Irish mental health policy, suicide (and to a lesser extent attempted suicide) has given rise to considerable public concern in recent years. This concern has been prompted by the sharp rise in the numbers of completed suicides reported over the past two decades as researchers and commentators attempt to find an explanation for this marked increase, particularly amongst young men. These trends are not, however, particular to Ireland as they reflect similar trends in international suicide statistics. Amongst the reasons proposed to explain these trends have been the rise of individualism, family breakdown, the loss of religious faith and community solidarity, substance abuse, unemployment or, conversely, 'Celtic Tiger' affluence. This chapter will examine Irish and international figures for fatal and non-fatal suicidal behaviour, placing them within an historical context. The wider social and public policy issues will be reviewed and some of the explanations put forward by recent research will be examined within the context of the significant gender differences in suicidal behaviour.

Definitions of suicidal behaviour

Suicide is both a personal tragedy and a social challenge and it is necessary when discussing statistics, trends and analyses to remember that each suicidal death is the end point of a painful personal struggle by the deceased which leaves the lives of the bereaved with difficult and complex grief. Definitions of suicide are complicated by the necessity of distinguishing between deaths which were intentionally fatal, those which were accidentally fatal (i.e. those who attempted to harm themselves but did not mean to die), those who intended to die but did not – often called 'failed suicides' and those who intended only to harm themselves – variously known as parasuicide, attempted suicide or, perhaps most accurately, deliberate self harm. What is sought in this terminology is the most appropriate way of including both intent and outcome. Perhaps the simplest definition of suicide is that which appears in the 1973 edition of the *Encyclopaedia Britannica* as 'the human act of self-inflicting one's own life cessation'. More recently, Canetto and Lester (1995: 6) have proposed using the outcome-based term 'fatal suicidal behaviour' for suicidal acts which end in death, and 'non-fatal suicidal behaviour' for suicidal actions that do not result in death. 'An advantage of this nomenclature is that it does not make assumptions about the suicidal person's intent'.

Current suicide statistics

Ireland

Prior to 1969 the Irish suicide rate was relatively stable and 1970 can be taken as the pivotal year in the rapid and prolonged increase in Irish suicide figures. Table 7.1 and figure 7.1 summarise these figures for the years 1970–2003. Table 7.1 shows an almost uninterrupted year-on year-increase in the overall figures for both sexes in this 34-year period, with the number in 2003 between eight and nine times what it was in 1970. It can also be seen that the rise in suicide mortality has been almost equally dramatic for both men and women – with almost a ninefold increase for men and over a tenfold increase for women in this period.

Between 1949 and 1969 the average overall suicide rate (i.e. suicide mortality per 100,000 of the population) was 2.39. However, as figure 7.1 shows, the rate rose from 2.6 for males in 1969 to 23.5 in 1998, falling to 19.2 in 2002. There was a similar upward, though not as dramatic, trend for females with the rates rising from 1.00 in 1969 to 5.1 in 1999 and falling to 4.1 in 2002.

As well as presenting a clear gender difference in completed suicide rates, Irish figures also display a marked age differential for fatal suicidal behaviour – both in general and between the sexes. Table 7.2 shows the rates for males and females for the 11 years from 1993 to 2003 by five-year age groups. It can be seen that for males the most common age group for completed suicides is 25 to 29 years, while for females it is 50 to 54 years. The National Suicide Review Group (2001: 21), in their in-depth analysis of the figures for 1997, found that females were significantly older than males when they engaged in fatal suicidal behaviour, with the mean age of females being 44.1 years and that for males 37.4 years.

Table 7.1 **Suicide mortality by sex 1970–2003 (Ireland)**

Year	Total	Males	Females
1970	52	44	8
1971	81	59	22
1972	90	65	25
1973	105	76	29
1974	118	92	26
1975	148	104	44
1976	183	129	54
1977	159	105	54
1978	163	106	57
1979	193	145	48
1980	216	143	73
1981	223	158	65
1982	241	178	63
1983	282	202	80
1984	232	164	68
1985	276	216	60
1986	283	217	66
1987	245	185	60
1988	266	195	71
1989	278	213	65
1990	334	251	83
1991	346	283	63
1992	363	304	59
1993	327	260	67
1994	395	305	90
1995	404	321	83
1996	409	435	64
1997	478	386	92
1998	514	433	81
1999	455	358	97
2000	486	395	91
2001	448	356	92
2002	451	371	80
2003	444	358	86

Source: CSO, Dept of Vital Statistics, 2004.

Figure 7.1 **Suicide rates (male, female and total population)**

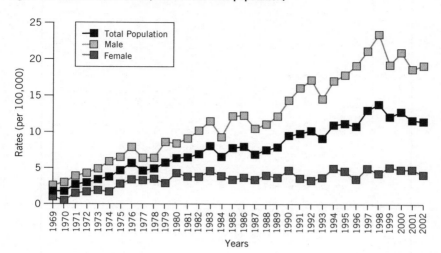

Source: CSO, Department of Vital Statistics, 2003.

It does not follow, however, that only young men are at high risk of suicide. 'Globally, suicide rates tend to increase with age' (DeLeo, 2002: 187) and this has traditionally been the case (Cantor, 2000). As the World Health Organisation's World Report pointed out, while the absolute number of suicide cases recorded is actually higher among those under 45 years of age than among those over 45 years, given demographic distributions, suicide rates are generally higher among older people. (WHO, 2002c: 187)

The figures in tables 7.1 and 7.2 suggest that the numbers of completed suicides in Ireland may in fact have peaked in 1998, when they reached a total of 514, falling by 13.6 per cent between 1998 and 2003. However, it is probably too soon to be certain whether the figures have stabilised at this rate or whether they will continue to fall.

Reliability

Much of the debate surrounding Ireland's suicide figures has centred on the reliability of the statistics, specifically on the under-reporting of suicide for cultural, legal and administrative reasons. The CSO uses the information provided by the Gardaí on Form 104 for classifying deaths as suicide. This form is used for supplementing the information on the Coroner's Certificate. Since the publication of the Report of the National Task Force on Suicide (Department of Health and Children, 1998b), Form 104 has been redrafted to provide more detailed information on the deceased. However, prior to 1993 suicide was a criminal offence under Irish law. Under the Coroner's Act, 1962,

Table 7.2 **Suicide rates 1993–2003 by age and gender**

5 Year	1993 M	1993 F	1994 M	1994 F	1995 M	1995 F	1996 M	1996 F	1997 M	1997 F	1998 M	1998 F	1999 M	1999 F	2000 M	2000 F	2001 M	2001 F	2002 M	2002 F	2003 M	2003 F
0–4	0	0	0	0	0	0	0	0	0	0	0	0	0	0	0	0	0	0	0	0	0	0
5–9	0	0	0	0	0.7	0	0	0	0	0	0	0	0	0	0	0	0	0	0	0	0	0
10–14	4.4	0	1.1	0	1.7	1.2	2.4	0	2.4	0	0.6	0.7	1.3	0.7	0.7	0	1.4	0	0	0	1.4	1.5
15–19	8.9	1.2	13	3.7	16.9	3.1	14.9	5.4	17	4.2	23.1	4.1	19.9	5.4	19.8	4.3	15.5	6.9	19	3.9	17.2	3.3
20–24	20.4	5.1	31.6	5	31.8	4.2	37.6	3.5	50.7	8.2	46.9	4.7	32.7	6.4	32.3	9.3	29.1	6.6	26.5	4.6	38.6	6.6
25–29	29.6	2.4	23.6	3.2	26.2	7.9	41	5.4	32.2	3.7	41.3	4.3	38.3	4.2	38.5	6	33.7	6.4	33.9	3.7	31.4	6.3
30–34	17.4	7.7	38.1	3.8	26.8	7.5	28.2	6	28.8	5.2	37.1	3	26.1	7.5	33.1	0.7	30.4	4.4	27.8	4.2	19.7	6.4
35–39	23.1	5.7	21.2	6.4	27.6	5.5	31.7	5.4	37	7.6	24	9	22.9	5.9	29.5	7.3	27.7	6.5	28.9	6.5	22.5	4.1
40–44	25.7	6.1	22.1	7.7	31.9	9.3	26.6	4.2	26.9	4.9	38	8	23.9	5.5	32.4	8.6	27.9	6.1	23	6.8	25.3	3.6
45–49	16.1	6.9	26.5	9.4	17.8	7.3	22	6.3	25.3	7.1	28.3	9.5	24.7	6	24.3	7.6	20.5	6.6	21	6.4	17.4	11.8
50–54	11.9	8.6	21.9	13.1	22.3	9.2	14.8	6.5	21.9	9.2	32.3	5.9	16.4	11.2	31.1	8.1	25.5	6.2	28	7.9	18.6	4.3
55–59	28.7	8.3	25.5	10.9	14.4	6.6	24.4	2.6	29.1	6.5	25.6	5	27.1	10.9	18.2	3.5	19.3	7.7	21.2	9.3	21.9	5.9
60–64	19.3	5.8	13.3	4.4	17.7	7.3	17.5	7.2	21.5	7.1	14.2	8.4	20.9	8.3	29.8	4	18.8	6.7	25.1	4	28.5	7.5
65–69	18.4	4.4	15.1	11.9	25.1	1.5	11.6	0	16.5	12.2	22.7	4.6	25.7	9.2	11.2	7.6	17.5	6	18.8	1.5	13.6	1.4
70–74	21.7	1.6	13.7	12.7	19.8	3.2	12	1.6	8	11.2	22.1	0	14.1	1.6	16	6.6	11.8	0	17.5	5	13.2	1.7
75–79	17.5	4.2	26.2	0	17.3	6.3	25.6	4.1	28.1	4	19.1	3.9	10.8	5.8	13.6	5.8	13.5	5.8	13.4	3.8	13.4	3.8
80–84	9.6	3.1	14.2	6	23.5	0	19	0	9.6	0	9.8	2.9	19.6	5.9	4.8	5.8	9.3	8.5	13.5	2.8	17.2	0
85+	0	0	10.8	4.5	30	0	18.9	0	0	4	16.5	3.8	23.8	0	7.7	0	0	0	14.1	0	0	3.4
ALL	14.6	3.7	17.1	5	17.9	4.6	19.2	3.5	21.2	5	23.5	4.3	19.3	5.1	21	4.8	18.7	4.8	19.2	4.1	18.1	4.3

Source: CSO, Department of Vital Statistics, 2004.

the duty of the Coroner is to enquire into all sudden, unexplained and unnatural deaths. Until 1984 some coroners recorded verdicts of death by suicide, even though under Section 30 of the 1962 Act, they were precluded from doing so as it states 'Questions of civil or criminal liability shall not be considered or investigated at an inquest'. As a result of the 1984 High Court case (McKeown and Scully), in which a widow challenged the verdict of a Coroner's Inquest, a verdict of suicide was no longer considered lawful.

However it was not only the secular law which led to the under-reporting of suicide. The Catholic Church (and other Christian faiths) views suicide as 'contrary to the will of a loving God' (Catholic Church, 1994: 491) and therefore a serious sin. This meant that until two or three decades ago, a suicide could not be buried in consecrated ground, thereby reinforcing the legal prohibition by prompting the bereaved to try to ensure that any conclusion other than suicide would be made about the death of their loved one.

Concerns that Irish suicide figures were unreliable for these legal and cultural reasons are perhaps now redundant. While Kelleher (1991) estimated that the official figures were between 15 per cent and 20 per cent lower than the actual figures, the extent of such discrepancies has been widely debated in Irish suicide literature. Cantor et al. (1997: 6) suggest that only a 'catastrophic' level of social change could have led to the reported increases in suicide figures between 1960 and 1989, and concluded that they must be due to 'substantial reporting and data collection influences'. In reply Kelleher et al. (1997: 17), having examined the relationship between accidental deaths and reported suicides, argued that 'under-reporting in Ireland was quite limited'. They also refer to the consistently lower suicide rates amongst Irish emigrants abroad in comparison with other ethnic groups and conclude that 'the rise in suicide in Ireland over the past three decades is genuine'. The recent findings of the National Suicide Review Group (2001) in this regard are reassuring. In their detailed study of all suicide deaths in every health board area in 1997 they found that there were 467 deaths. The CSO figure for the same year, using their standardised methods (see above) was 478. This suggests that the CSO figures for recent years can be relied on not to underestimate the real suicide mortality rates.

International comparisons

Suicide was the thirteenth leading cause of death worldwide in 2002, when an estimated 815,000 people took their own lives. This represents an annual global mortality rate of about 14.5 per 100,000 population – equivalent to one death every 40 seconds (DeLeo et al., 2002: 185).

Just as historical comparisons are difficult because of changes in recording procedures over the years, comparisons between countries are complicated by the variations in the way in which deaths are recorded. Despite these difficulties the World Health Organisation concludes that the relative ranking of national suicide rates is reasonably accurate (DeLeo et al., 2002: 189).

Table 7.3 **Age-adjusted suicide rates by country (most recent year available*)**

Country	Year	Total	Male: Female ratio
Australia	1998	17.9	4.1:1
Austria	1999	20.9	3.2:1
Brazil	1995	6.3	4.1:1
Canada	1997	15.0	3.9:1
China†	1999	18.3	1.0:1
Colombia	1995	4.5	4.1:1
Finland	1998	28.4	3.9:1
France	1998	20.0	3.2:1
Germany	1999	14.3	3.3:1
Greece	1998	4.2	3.7:1
Ireland	1997	16.8	4.3:1
Netherlands	1999	11.0	2.1:1
Norway	1997	14.6	2.7:1
Portugal	1999	5.4	3.8:1
Russian Federation	1998	43.1	6.2:1
Spain	1998	8.7	3.8:1
Sweden	1996	15.9	2.5:1
United Kingdom	1999	9.2	3.8:1
United States	1998	13.7	4.4:1
Ireland	2002	11.6	4.7:1

Source: Adapted from World Report on Violence and Health (WHO, 2002)
* 1997 Figures for Ireland included as on original report. CSO figures for 2002 included at end of table for comparison.
† Selected urban and rural areas. Excludes Hong Kong SAR.

Table 7.3 shows the suicide rates for a selected number of European and non-European countries for both men and women as reported to the World Health Organisation. The report points out that the highest suicide rates are found in Eastern Europe, for example the Russian Federation has a rate of 43.1, while Latin American countries have much lower rates, for example Colombia's rate is 4.5 and Brazil's is 6.3. Within Europe, Finland has the highest rate at 28.4 while Greece would appear to have the lowest rate in the European Union, at 4.2. Using the 1997 figures, Ireland would appear to be midway in these rankings, at 16.8. As Cantor (2000: 11) noted, in commenting on the stability of the rank order of national suicide rates over time, 'suicide rates are determined by persisting cross-national differences, including traditions, customs, religions, social attitudes and climate'.

The male/female ratio is positive in all countries, though it varies between 1.00: 1 in China to 6.2: 1 in the Russian Federation, suggesting that culturally defined gender roles and expectations may be important variables both across and within different societies in understanding gender differences in suicide figures. In Ireland the male/female ratio, at 4.7: 1 (in 2002), is amongst the highest in Europe, second only to the Russian Federation. In a survey of 22 Western nations, Ireland had the highest male: female differential, but this was 'driven more by relatively low female rates than by high male rates' (Cantor, 2000: 16).

Suicide rates are generally higher among older people, and this holds true for both men and women. The WHO global figures demonstrate this quite clearly. While Ireland is unusual with a primary peak in the 25–34 male age group (seen in table 7.2), in general, suicide rates among those aged 75 years and over are approximately three times higher than those in the 15–24 age group (DeLeo et al., 2002: 189).

Ireland is also within general, though not universal, European trends in the rise in its suicide rates over time. During the twentieth century, Finland, the Netherlands, Norway, Scotland, Spain and Sweden also experienced a significant increase in suicide mortality. However, England and Wales, Italy, New Zealand and Switzerland experienced a significant drop (DeLeo et al., 2002: 187). In the case of England and Wales, however, Gunnell et al. (2003: 165) suggest that changes in the toxicity of domestic gas and car exhaust fumes have contributed to this drop.

Non-fatal suicidal behaviour

The terms attempted suicide, parasuicide, deliberate self harm and non-fatal suicidal behaviour are often used interchangeably to describe the actions of an individual who inflicts harm on him or herself but which do not result in death. The intention of the person engaging in this behaviour is what distinguishes a 'failed' suicide event from an 'attempted suicide'. The National Parasuicide Registry describes parasuicide as 'any non fatal act which an individual deliberately undertakes knowing that it may cause them physical harm or even death'. (2001: vi) The first and second annual reports of the National Parasuicide Registry (2001; 2002), based on records of admissions to Accident and Emergency Departments in each health board area of the Republic of Ireland, provides the most comprehensive data on non-fatal suicidal behaviour ever compiled in Ireland. The 2002 report estimates that there were 10,537 attendances for suicidal behaviour involving 8,421 individuals and suggests that there has been an increase in all hospitals which returned data for the 2001 report (which included only four health boards). The 2002 figures show that the overall age-standardised rate of parasuicide was 167 per 100,000 for men and 237 per 100,000 women, giving a 42 per cent higher rate for females. The age specific rate for women peaked in the 15–19 age group while that for men peaked in the 20–24 age group. In contrast to the figures for completed suicides discussed above, women significantly exceeded men in almost all age groups; for example the female rate for the 10–19 age group was more than double the male rate. The only exception to this was in the 25–34 year age group where there were almost equal numbers of episodes by men and women. (National Parasuicide Registry, 2002: 115). The rates in the 25–34 year group were somewhat similar, but the female/male differential increased again in the 35–54 age group. From age 55 upwards, the rates in both men and women were relatively low.

Figure 7.2 **Attempted suicide episodes, 2002**

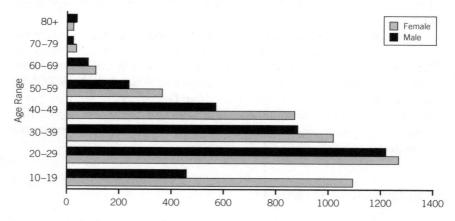

Source: Adapted from the Report of the National Parasuicide Registry Ireland, 2002.

This gender and age imbalance reflects international trends in non-fatal suicidal behaviour which as a general rule show that rates tend to be 2-3 times higher for women (with the exception of Finland) (DeLeo, 2002: 191). Data from the ongoing, cross national study of non-fatal suicidal behaviour in 13 countries show that in the majority of centres the highest rates were also found in the younger age groups and as in Ireland, the most common method used being overdosing, followed by cutting.

It is impossible to make any historical comparisons of parasuicide figures given the dearth of information available prior to the setting up of the Parasuicide Registry. What is interesting to note are the findings for 'Recommended Next

Care' in the report. Overall, within all health boards, almost three quarters (70.7 per cent) of all episodes led to a recommendation for admission, with the majority being admitted to a general ward. This contrasts with the findings of a year-long study in a large Dublin Accident and Emergency Department ten years previously (Allen and Cronin, 1992) which found that only 41 per cent of deliberate self-harm patients were admitted as in-patients to either a general or psychiatric hospital. This change may be due to the greater seriousness with which parasuicide admissions are now seen within the general medical service as a result of a decade of research, policy, training initiatives and increased resources.

Legislative, research and policy initiatives

Legislation

From the early 1990s the growing concern in many sectors of Irish society about increasing suicide rates led to a number of public policy initiatives. The first of these was the enactment of the Criminal Law (Suicide) Act 1993 which decriminalised suicide and attempted suicide. The decriminalisation of suicide did not, however, automatically lead to coroners being free to return verdicts of suicide. As a result of High and Supreme Court decisions, uncertainty still remained regarding the jurisdiction of the coroner in returning verdicts at inquest. In the case of Greene and McLoughlin (1995), a verdict was overturned on appeal to the High Court as the possibility of suicide was implied in the verdict of the coroner's jury. The appeal to the Supreme Court was dismissed on the grounds that the jury went outside its jurisdiction to inquire into what gave rise to the injury which resulted in death (Department of Justice, Equality and Law Reform, 2000). Because of this continuing confusion in the finding of verdicts of suicide the Task Force called for a review of the Coroner's Act 1962. This review, published in 2000, recommended that 'the jurisdiction of the coroner should include the investigation not only of the medical cause of death but also the investigation of the circumstances surrounding the death. This should be expressed in positive terms in the new Coroners Act' (no. 49). In recommendation no. 51 it stated specifically that 'suicide verdicts should be returned whenever it has been established beyond a reasonable doubt that a person has taken their own life' (Department of Justice, Equality and Law Reform, 2000: 63).

National Task Force on Suicide

The report of the National Task Force on Suicide (Department of Health and Children, 1998b) can be regarded as the blueprint for a National Suicide Prevention/Reduction Strategy. Its recommendations included the provision of training in the management of suicidal behaviour for all relevant personnel (e.g. medical and nursing staff, gardaí, coroners, prison staff, teachers); the establishment by each health board of a directory of appropriate voluntary and statutory services which should be available to the public; the provision of appropriate mental health care for prisoners; the provision of suicide prevention programmes in schools and within youth services and access to appropriate support and counselling services for young people; greater awareness of depression and its attendant risk of suicide amongst the elderly; support and training for those traumatised by suicidal behaviour and ongoing research and evaluation of these and other initiatives.

Administrative changes

Form 104, used by the Gardai and the Central Statistics Office to record suicidal deaths, was redrafted on the recommendation of the Task Force to include the social and personal circumstances of each case of suicide, in order to facilitate a better understanding of the causes of suicide (Department of Health and Children, 1998b: 24).

The Task Force's recommendation that the 'availability of medicines harmful in overdose be restricted' (1998b: 48) was implemented with the introduction of the Statutory Instrument (no. 150) 2001: Medicinal Products (Control of Paracetamol) Regulations. The regulations restrict the maximum pack sizes of paracetamol when sold in pharmacies and supermarkets, demands the use of blister packaging, and prohibits the sale of more than one pack in a single transaction. It also requires suitable labelling warning of the dangers of overdoses. It is hoped that these restrictions will discourage the use of this potentially dangerous product by those engaged in self-harming behaviour.

Suicide research

In November 1995, the Suicide Research Foundation (NSRF) was founded in Cork by the late Dr Michael Kelleher. The aims of the Foundation, which is an independent research body in receipt of government funding, are to define the true extent of suicidal behaviour and to develop strategies for its prevention. At the request of the Department of Health and Children, the National Parasuicide Registry was set up by the NSRF.

Following the recommendation of the second Report of the National Task Force (Department of health and Children, 1998b) a National Suicide Review Group was set up by the chief executives of the health boards. Their extensive national study (referred to above) was published in 2001. This report reinforces the recommendations of the National Task Force as well as providing a detailed and up-to-date demographic analysis of fatal and non-fatal suicidal behaviour in Ireland.

Suicide in prisons

Both the National Task Force Report (Department of Health and Children, 1998b) and the 1999 Report of the Advisory Group on Prison Deaths (Department of Justice, Equality and Law Reform, 1999a) examined the particular concerns raised by the suicide and attempted suicide of those in custody. In 1996 a National Steering Group on Deaths in Prisons was appointed to review the recommendations made in the 1991 Advisory Group's report. Their report (Department of Justice, Equality and Law Reform, 1999a) found that between 1991 and 1997, 41 prisoners took their own lives in Irish prisons. Reviewing the 57 recommendations of the 1991 Report, they concluded that 34 of the 1991 recommendations had been implemented in full, 15 had been partially implemented and eight were not implemented at all (1999a: 23). Suicide awareness groups have been established in each prison to progress and monitor the implementation of procedures and training to reduce deaths in custody. All new prison officers receive training in suicide awareness and in some prisons there is a special telephone facility to enable offenders to contact the Samaritans if they wish. However, the Review Group was not satisfied with the facilities for psychiatrically ill patients, and suggested that 'a high support facility be provided in each closed institution for offenders exhibiting suicidal tendencies' (1999a: 35).

Suicide and sexual orientation

International studies have been consistent in finding a strong correlation between homosexuality and suicidal behaviour. The United States Surgeon General's Report on Youth Suicide concluded that gay youth are at a particularly increased risk for attempted and completed suicide. In an innovative US study involving male twins, researchers found a fourfold increase in suicidal ideation among the twins reporting same gender sexual orientation, and they were over six times more likely to have actually attempted suicide (Herrell et al., 1999). Similar figures emerged from a 21-year longitudinal study in New Zealand, where gay, lesbian and bisexual young people were also found to have been six times more likely to attempt suicide. (Ferguson et al., 1999). Of recent Irish reports, however, only the National Suicide Review Group (2001) makes any recommendations which refer specifically to this vulnerable group of young people.

Gender and suicide: a dilemma for young men

The two main questions thrown up by even a cursory assessment of the Irish and international statistics outlined above are 'Why are more people taking their own lives now than thirty years ago?' and 'Why are men more likely to engage in fatal suicidal behaviour and women in non-fatal suicidal behaviour?'

These questions are interlinked as the explanations proposed for the former very often contribute to greater contradictions regarding the latter. A number of Irish researchers have proposed reasons for these rises in Irish figures. Kelleher (1996) suggested that the factors which contributed to social 'anomie' – decline in religious practice, changes in family life (the rise in non-marital births, increasing break up of relationships etc.), the increasing use of alcohol and illicit drugs – have contributed to this rise and that young boys are disproportionately affected by these changes. Kelleher et al. (1997: 15) have postulated that the increasing number of women in third-level education and the fact that 'female students are outperforming their male counterparts' may be contributing factors. Depression and mental illness have been consistently linked to fatal suicidal behaviour (Lonnqvist, 2000: 108). International studies have consistently shown, however, that despite their higher incidence and prevalence of affective disorders, women have substantially lower suicide rates (Murphy, 2000: 138). This presents the dilemma as to why these female psychiatric morbidity rates do not translate into higher suicide rates. It has been suggested that women's choice of less lethal methods of self-harm results in greater numbers of attempted suicides but fewer completed suicides. This explanation is essentially tauto-logical and presents us with two problems: firstly it assumes that attempted suicides are primarily failed suicides because insufficient lethality was employed; and secondly, that more lethal methods of self-harm are not available to women. Neither of these assumptions is supported by recent evidence. The Parasuicide Registry figures for 2001 (National Parasuicide Registry, 2002) show that both men and women used overdoses as the primary method of self-harm, with cutting being the second major method used. Only 4.6 per cent of parasuicide episodes involved poisoning, hanging or drowning, though men were more likely to employ these methods (National Parasuicide Registry, 2002: P.IE-7). The 2002 figures show a similar pattern, with 63.9 per cent of male and 78.4 per cent of female episodes involving overdoses (National Parasuicide Registry, 2003: 119). The figures for completed suicides in 2001 show a similar convergence; 70.8 per cent of cases for men and 62.2 per cent for women employed either drowning or hanging (P.ie-17). These figures do not suggest a sufficiently greater preference for, or the restriction of, more lethal methods to men. Fatal actions such as drowning and hanging are as available to women as to men. This therefore still leaves us with the question, 'Why do more men take their own lives?'

Canetto and Lester (1995), while querying the gendered assumptions made when distinguishing between fatal and non-fatal suicidal behaviour, raise the question of traditional role expectations in our attitudes to attempted and fatal suicides. They suggest that there may be some 'nexus between conforming to traditional feminine roles and low rates of suicidal behaviour in women as killing oneself is viewed as masculine. Attempting, but not "succeeding" at suicide, on the other hand, meshes with traditional expectations of women' (1995: 27).

While all acts of suicide have a composite of contributing factors and are rooted in hopelessness and despair, suicide can be described as the ultimate violence one can inflict on oneself. Perhaps therefore a useful avenue to explore in trying to understand these gender differences would be to examine the role that violence and risk taking play in the social construction of young men's identity and self-esteem.

Alcohol misuse has been recognised as being closely associated with both violence and suicidal behaviour (Murphy, 2000; McEvoy and Richardson, 2004). There is rising public concern about the numbers of assaults and homicides on city streets involving almost exclusively young men who have been drinking heavily. Kerkhof (2003) suggests that, psychologically speaking, alcohol misuse and suicidal behaviour are the same. The traditional cultural constriction of emotional expression by young men, making them seem 'invulnerable to themselves and to others' (Smyth et al., 2003) adds to the 'perilousness' of the male experience. Studies by McKeon and Carrick (1991) and Gavigan and McKeon (1995) found that young men were significantly less likely to attend their general practitioner for help with psychological problems and more likely to regard those suffering from depression as feeling sorry for themselves. Added to this is the extra danger of risk taking behaviour which is evidenced in the numbers of young men involved in serious and fatal car accidents. The Report on Men's Health in Ireland (McEvoy and Richardson, 2004) shows recent Irish figures on these aspects of men's risk taking behaviours, which reinforce 'their exposure to illness and accidental deaths' (2004: 7). In reflecting on these gender differences in suicidal behaviour, Kelleher (1996: 49) quotes a colleague who suggested that 'in harsher and less settled times, such young men might have been at the forefront in wartime situations, where risk taking is both institutionalised and rewarded by hero status'.

This combination of factors raises the spectre of a compulsory 'macho' male identity being demanded of young men. Those who are, or appear to be, less 'macho' or who may fit the 'gay man' stereotype of gentleness and sensitivity, are more likely to be bullied and intimidated and this can demand of them compensatory aggressive and risk-taking behaviour. In this way violence is a 'resource for the construction of masculinity' (Hearn, 1998: 216).

The implications of this association of aggression and risk taking with a normative masculine identity in modern Irish culture may be proving lethal for young men, interacting as it does with other social and personal stressors such as alcohol, drug use, depression and mental illness.

Directions for change

Even if, as the current figures tentatively suggest, the Irish suicide rate has peaked, it is still unacceptably high. There have been a number of important Irish research and policy initiatives which have examined the extent of, and the possible reasons for, these high rates of suicidal behaviour. Numerous recommendations have been made in official reports and many have been implemented. However, there are still a number of areas where policy and practice may be failing to support those most at risk of self-directed violence. Education and awareness programmes in schools and colleges have been recommended as a means of reaching young people who are at great risk of suicidal behaviour (Aware, 1998; Department of Health and Children, 1998b). Despite these recommendations and the growing acceptance that the con-struction of masculinity in our culture may be an important contributory factor in our young male suicide rates (see, for example, Smyth et al., 2003), pro-grammes to address this, such as Exploring Masculinities, have met with serious resistance from both the media and the educational system itself. Smyth et al. (2003) in their analysis of this resistance found that even where the programme is in use in boys' schools, the sections dealing with sexual orientation and violence against women and children are usually omitted. Such widespread avoidance of these critical public policy issues cannot but reinforce the very cultural pressures which may lead some young men and women to self-harm and suicide. The current update of the programme is a welcome development but it may still face resistance and selective implementation.

While there may not be consensus about the exact role that mental illness plays in suicidal behaviour (see for example Kelleher et al., 1997; Casey, 2003; Smyth et al., 2003), there is agreement that the provision of accessible psychiatric and psychological services is an essential ingredient in the reduction of suicide mortality. The lack of such services has been highlighted by the report on Child and Adolescent Services (Department of Health and Children, 2001a) which found a large discrepancy between the required numbers of appropriate inpatient beds and those currently available. Commenting on this gap in services, the Irish College of Psychiatrists considers that 'existing Child Psychiatry is not equipped to deal with the older adolescent age group'. Neither the Mental Health Act 2001, nor the government's health strategy document *Quality and Fairness: A Health System For You* (Department of Health and Children, 2001b) adequately addresses this worrying gap in service provision. These difficulties, at the level of service provision and in the wider society where identity is shaped and supported, present major challenges to efforts to tackle the health problem that suicidal behaviour presents in contemporary Irish life.

Further reading

Smyth, C., MacLachlan, M. and Clare, A. (2003) *Cultivating Suicide: Destruction of Self in a Changing Ireland.* Dublin: Liffey.

Hawton, K. and Van Heeringen, K. (eds) *The International Handbook of Suicide and Attempted Suicide.* Chichester: Wiley.

DeLeo, D., Bertolote, J., and Lester, D. (2003) 'Self-directed violence', in

Krug, E. G. et al. (eds), *World Report on Violence and Health.* Geneva: WHO.

Department of Health and Children (1998b) *Report of the National Task Force on Suicide.* Dublin: Stationery Office.

Chapter 8

Women and mental health

Patricia Kennedy
Elizabeth Hickey

Introduction

This chapter explores mental health from a women's perspective. Historically women who did not conform to social norms were defined as 'mad' or 'bad' and concepts such as hysteria, penis envy and castration complex (Mitchell, 1975) have been used to explain women's behaviour. This chapter focuses on the link between women's mental health and cultural and socio-economic factors such as poverty, discrimination, domestic violence, the dual burden of caring and earning, and sex-role stereotyping. It focuses on how women's mental health problems have been linked in public discourse to their reproductive role and in particular to pre-menstrual syndrome (PMS), post-natal depression, abortion and the menopause. It focuses particularly on depression, as this is the most common type of mental disorder experienced by women (table 8.1). It presents a blueprint for a woman friendly mental health service and recommendations on how to tackle the structural causes of women's depression.

Gender aspects of mental health

There are gender differences in the frequency, clinical expression and outcome of mental illness (Kohen, 2003). While mental health is a concern for men and women, the experience of both has been different in terms of discourse and responses. Kohen (2003) suggests that the most important gender issues in mental health are: epidemiological differences between the sexes; social concomitants of mental health problems and mental health problems exclusive to women.

In general, gender stereotyping occurs in medicine. Traditionally women's health has been viewed in a narrow physiological context in relation to reproductive health (Ussher, 1992; Doyal, 1995 and in the Irish context by Murphy-Lawless, 2002). Women experience certain disorders more commonly than men, especially depression and anxiety related disorders. Alcoholism, substance misuse and anti-social personality are more common in men (Rhodes and Goering, 1998; Weissmann et al., 1993). In Ireland, statistics relating to mental illness are incomplete. There is an over-reliance on in-patient data focusing on treatment and admissions to psychiatric hospitals and units with a lack of substantial community-based research. Prior (1999) discusses the inadequacies of traditional attempts to measure mental disorder suggesting that 'any measurement of the extent of mental disorder should include but not be confined to mental health service users' (1999: 15). Official statistics (Department of Health and Children, 2003a) show that more men than women are admitted to psychiatric hospitals. The epidemiology of mental illness is quite different for men and women. Because of the relative frequency of depression among the female population, we are focusing primarily on depression while discussing some other mental disorders.

Depression

Depressive illness includes major depression, dysthymic disorder (a less severe type of depression) and bi-polar mood disorder. Researchers and mental health practitioners have repeatedly identified depression as a problem that particularly affects women (Stoppard, 2000). Internationally it is the most common mental health problem for which women are hospitalised, with women outnumbering men by three to one (Busfield, 1996; McGrath et al., 1990). In the US, women are three times more likely than men to be prescribed antidepressant medication (Baum et al., 1998). Statistics from the US show that nearly twice as many women (12 per cent) as men (6.6 per cent) suffer from depressive illness (Regier et al., 1993).

The gender difference in depression is not seen until after adolescence and decreases again at the menopause (Stoppard, 2000). Physiological factors are often given as the explanation for this. However, other factors such as women's multiple roles, or increased risk of violence and poverty have been cited as contributing to the statistical difference. In Ireland, more women than men are admitted to psychiatric hospitals and units as a result of depressive illness as indicated in table 8.1

When used to describe a mood, the word 'depression' refers to feelings of sadness, despair and discouragement. Depression may thus be a normal state of feelings, which any person can experience from time to time. 'Depression' is also a clinical and scientific term, which may refer to a 'symptom' seen in a variety of mental or physical disorders, or it may refer to a 'mental disorder' itself. The Diagnostic and Statistical Manual of Mental Disorders, DSM-IV, which is the internationally recognised standard for the diagnosis of mental disorders, classifies depression by severity, recurrence, and association with

Table 8.1 **Irish psychiatric hospitals and units: admissions by diagnosis and gender for selected diagnoses, 1997–2000**

Year	Depressive disorders Male	Depressive disorders Female	Personality disorders Male	Personality disorders Female	Neuroses Male	Neuroses Female
1997	2,772	4,133	670	701	643	875
1998	2,973	4,341	598	727	681	975
1999	3,096	4,221	611	722	623	868
2000	3,148	4,382	549	624	539	851

Source: Compiled by the authors from *Health Statistics, 2002*. Department of Health and Children (2003a).

mania (American Psychiatric Association, 1994; Stotland, 2004). Depression is a common mental disorder, which comes in many different forms, from mild to severe. It is characterised by low mood, hopelessness, dejection, pessimistic thoughts, loss of energy, lack of interest in activities usually engaged in, social withdrawal, various bodily complaints, aches and pains, feelings of anxiety. People may suffer from sleeplessness, or oversleeping, lack of appetite or over-eating. In some cases there may be suicidal thoughts or actions (Stoppard, 2000).

Why does depression occur?
Theories to explain depression cover a wide spectrum including biological, psychological and social. While in recent years there has been a shift away from the notion of one single cause to the idea of a multi-factorial approach, different disciplines continue to stress a particular approach over another (Stoppard, 2000). Biological explanations tend to dominate within the psychiatric model. Bourne (1998) warns against the current tendency to oversimplify the causes of mental illness by proposing a 'single cause theory'. According to him, single cause theories give rise to what he describes as the 'biological fallacy' and the 'psychological fallacy' in which a mental disorder is attributed solely to either a biological or psychological cause. Busfield (1996) also discusses the limitations of a medical model, especially its narrowly based biological orientation and its separation of individuals from their environment and their particular life circumstances.

Physiological models of depression
In physiological models of depression, emphasis is placed on genetics and biochemistry as causes of depression (Paykel, 1991). Traditionally, there has been a focus on women's hormones as having a strong role in determining moods and being implicated in reproductive syndromes such as PMS, post-natal depression (PND) and menopausal problems (Bebbington, 1996; Gallant

and Derry, 1995). However, this research has been severely criticised (Ussher, 2000). Stoppard (2000), while agreeing that there is little evidence for seeing depression in purely physiological terms, cautions against ignoring the body, as fundamentally depression is an embodied experience. She suggests that non-medical researchers have neglected the body in their study of depression. She gives two possible explanations for this, first that non-medical researchers are anxious to emphasise the psychological and sociological influences, which they believe have been ignored by the medical profession. Second, she sees researchers as having more difficulty integrating knowledge about the body with more subjective psychological and sociological knowledge (Stoppard, 2000: 13).

Psychosocial explanations
In recent years there has been a move away from purely physiological explanations with an increased acknowledgement of psychosocial factors. Referred to as the 'diathesis-stress model' (Stoppard, 2000; Champion and Power, 1995), it proposes that if an individual has certain underlying personal vulnerabilities, and then is exposed to stressful life experiences, that person is under increased likelihood of becoming depressed. It has been suggested that the socialisation process which encourages feminine traits such as dependency and care giving in women is possibly making women more vulnerable to depression (Stoppard, 2000). This approach is gender specific and looks to women's psychological make up in its attempts to identify the causes of depression in women (Stoppard, 2000).

From this perspective, the importance that women place on their relationships to give them a coherent sense of self is emphasised. This approach, based on the work of Gilligan (1982) and Miller (1986), emphasises positive qualities such as nurturance and caring. When these qualities are not valued, as is often the case in the modern patriarchal society, it may lead to depression in women. Stoppard (2000) has also identified the centrality of women's relationships to their psychological well-being and has posited that when there are difficulties in this regard that it can lead to depression.

Multiple-role strain
The difficulties of combining multiple roles – worker outside the home, wife, mother, carer as well as an unequal burden of domestic duties – have been cited as one of the factors that contribute to the higher rates of mental health problems in women (Bebbington, 1996; Doyal, 1995; Kennedy, 2002). In a review of the literature, Ussher (2000: 79) summarises the social and environmental factors associated with higher rates of mental health problems as: marital status, caring roles, employment status, gender role socialisation, representations of femininity, multiple role strain and conflict and sexual violence.

The UK Department of Health Consultation document on mental health care for women, *Women's Mental Health: Into the Mainstream* (UK Department of Health, 2002: 9), identified a number of groups of women who may be particularly vulnerable to mental ill health:

- Women who are mothers and carers
- Older women
- Women from black and minority ethnic groups
- Lesbian and bisexual women
- Transsexual women
- Women involved in prostitution
- Women offenders
- Women with learning disabilities
- Women who abuse alcohol and drugs

There has been no substantial research focusing specifically on the mental health needs of women in Ireland. However, according to *Perspectives on the Provision of Counselling for Women in Ireland* (Batt et al., 2003), women are particularly unhappy with the current mental health services and feel that in the absence of counselling and other organised responses to their distress, their problems are being medicalised. The Women's Health Council has commissioned research on the gender aspect of mental health policy and services which will be launched in 2005 as *Women's Mental Health: Promoting a Gendered Approach to Policy and Service Provision.*

Women in Ireland: the social context

In the Women's Health Council report (NWCI, 2002: 19) *Promoting Women's Health: A Population Investment for Ireland's Future,* it is argued that:

> inequalities exist in relation to health in Irish society, those who live in poverty are subject to poorer or bad health, and women have a critical influence in relation to family and social support as well as to their own direct health needs.

This is in line with literature which links women's social disadvantage with poor health. In Ireland, women are at a higher risk of poverty than men (NWCI, 2003). Households headed by someone working full time in the home form the largest income poverty group (NWCI, 2003). Households headed by a person over 65 are also at greater risk of poverty, again predominantly women (NWCI, 2003). Poverty is not only the absence of income and physical resources but also means exclusion from participation in society, lack of power and the unequal distribution of resources. Coakley highlights the incredible stress experienced by women and particularly mothers living on a low income in Ireland (2004a, 2004b). They find themselves in a position in which they are in a constant struggle to obtain nutritious food and other material resources on behalf of their families. Lack of childcare facilities, and lack of financial supports to pay for childcare are the biggest barriers to women's participation in employment, education and training. Kennedy (2004) highlights the wage differential between men and women. The NWCI (2004) indicates that the gap between the average hourly rate for men and women is currently 15 per cent. They suggest that women's absence from paid employment for caring responsibilities is the main reason for this. Women tend to be concentrated in the low paid, lower level positions in employment and are more likely than men to be in part-time work. Kennedy (2002, 2004) has written extensively on the link between reproduction, caring and earning a living and the burden this places on Irish women.

In *Women, Disadvantage and Health* (Women's Health Council, 2004) the link between socio-economic status and health is outlined. Women do not form a homogeneous group and certain women are more likely to experience disadvantage than others. These include carers, women with disabilities, older women, Traveller women and asylum seeking and refugee women.

Intimate violence

Stotland (2004: 2) indicates that victims of domestic violence (an estimated 8–17 per cent of all women in the US each year) are at increased risk of mental health problems. The World Health Organisation (Watts and Zimmerman, 2002) in a review of over 50 population-based studies of the prevalence of domestic violence estimates that between 10 and 50 per cent of women who have had partners have been physically assaulted. An Irish study reports that 39 per cent of women who have been in intimate relationships reported having experienced violence (Bradley et al., 2002). According to Bradley et al. (2002) there is a high correlation between domestic violence and anxiety and depression. In several studies from around the world women who were being abused were found to have more depression symptoms than other non-battered women. Similarly, Heath (2001) suggests that there is a high incidence of depression and psychiatric disorders, self-harm, drug and alcohol abuse as well as anxiety disorders including Post Traumatic Stress Disorder (PTSD), eating disorders, substance abuse and suicide among those who have experienced domestic violence. Several studies have shown that women are at greater risk than men of childhood sexual abuse, domestic violence, rape and sexual assault (Koss et al., 1994; European Women's Lobby, 1999). In particular, childhood sexual abuse has been associated with women's vulnerability to depression (Stoppard, 2000). Physical and sexual abuse by a male partner in intimate relationships has also been linked to the increased incidence of depression in women (McGrath et al., 1990).

Romito and Guerin (2000) suggest that many women presenting at the emergency room with physical injuries are redirected to the psychological and psychiatric services. They are treated for their distressing symptoms with medication, without any exploration of the violence that they were suffering at the hands of their partners. In Ireland, a national study of Irish experiences, beliefs and attitudes concerning sexual violence (the SAVI study) indicated that one quarter of women subjected to sexual violence reported symptoms consistent with PTSD (McGee et al., 2002).

Women's specific mental health problems

Hoffman and Massion (2000: 3) refer to how 'all our health care systems are built around an outdated concept of women's lives. Today's professional medicine took form in the mid-nineteenth century, when women were considered "bodies built around a uterus"'. There are physiological differences between men's and women's bodies and as a result there are certain experiences, including menstruation, childbirth and abortion that only women can experience. It is to the link between these experiences and mental health that attention is now turned.

Pre-menstrual tension

Stoppard (2000: 126) reviews literature on young women's expressed experiences of the menarche and concludes they often report feelings of embarrassment, shame and secrecy. At the same time, first menstruation is often seen as a rite of passage and the beginning of womanhood. It is in this social and cultural context that premenstrual tension syndrome (PMS) must be understood. Defined in DSM-IV (American Psychiatric Association, 1994) as Premenstrual Dysphoric Disorder (PMDD), three to four per cent of women report premenstrual mood changes and physical symptoms that interfere with their work and social life.

Post-natal depression

The months following the birth of a baby are a particularly vulnerable time for women. Levy et al. (1993: 148) refer to the maternity blues as the 'brief period of emotional lability affecting approximately 60 per cent of women in the first week of the puerperium' and conclude that it would appear to be a normal condition on a worldwide scale, judging by the incidence of the syndrome. It manifests itself in crying, anxiety, tiredness, confusion, restlessness, lack of concentration, anorexia, forgetfulness and insomnia in the three to four days following delivery. A more serious psychological condition is postnatal depression, with up to ten per cent of women developing it and, more seriously, postpartum psychosis, which occur in 0.1 per cent of all births. Both of these conditions have serious health implications not only for the woman but also for her baby (UK Department of Health, 2002; Kennedy, 2002). Ball (1994) indicates that there are various factors associated with postnatal depression. These include obstetric problems, often linked to dissatisfaction with the management of childbirth, poor relationship/separation from own mother, unplanned pregnancy, marital conflict, lack of a confidante, life events in year preceding pregnancy, social class and social problems. In Ireland, postnatal depression is viewed primarily as a medical problem but research tends to indicate that while there is a medical basis to some types of depression, the condition can be very strongly related to social circumstances and in particular to lack of social support (Enkin et al., 1995). The Post Natal Depression Association of Ireland (PNDAI) (Pigot, 1996) outlines a suggested post-natal depression policy, indicating that what is needed is for statutory and voluntary organisations and maternity services to work together to provide greater levels of support for women sufferers and their families. The PNDAI views a mother's experience of postnatal depression in the context of her role as carer, as earner as well as life giver:

> The pressure to go back to work or to stay away from work are equally damaging to a mother's mental health after having a baby. We must work towards more economic and social support for mothers as they face the conflicting dilemmas which motherhood can bring . . . post-natal distress is not simply a woman's complaint. We must recognise the pain and distress that it causes to partners, families and friends. We all need greater education and a more realistic attitude to childbirth and parenting. All mothers deserve support. (Pigot, 1996: 72)

Post Abortion Syndrome

Handy (1982) reviews the literature concerning psychological and social aspects of induced abortion. Although some women experience adverse psychological effects, the great majority do not. In contrast, refused abortion can result in psychological distress and an impoverished environment for the offspring. Arthur (1997) argues that 'over the last decade, a general consensus has been reached in the medical and scientific communities that most women who have abortions experience little or no psychological harm' (1997: 1). Discussions about the psychosocial and emotional aspects of abortion is dominated by whether or not there exits what has been defined as Post Abortion Syndrome (PAS). This syndrome has been put forward as a type of Post Traumatic Stress Disorder (PTSD) whose sufferers experience symptoms similar to those experienced by Vietnam Veterans. Dr Vincent Rue is accredited with introducing the subject of PAS. In the 1980s he gave several papers at conferences organised by anti-abortion organisations, in which he argued that abortion can lead to PAS

(Lee, 2001: 10). Rue developed diagnostic criteria, listing symptoms as including helplessness, hopelessness, sadness, sorrow, lowered self-esteem, distrust, regret, relationship disruption, communication impairment and/or restriction and self-condemnation (Rue, 1995: 20). Lee (2001) argues that the British based 'Life' organisation suggests that PAS exists and that the symptoms include grief, guilt and shame, anger, self-pity, depression, moodiness, crying, drug taking, overeating, going off food, having nightmares, sleeplessness, going off sex, having a lot of sex and disliking oneself. Lee suggests that this extensive list 'is put forward as characteristic of PAS because of course, the broader the set of symptoms becomes, the easier it becomes to argue that women suffer from PAS' (2001: 11).

In May 1990, a panel from the American Psychiatric Association argued that there is no evidence to support PAS and that restrictions on access to abortion by Government are more harmful (Lee, 2003). The Royal College of Obstetrics and Gynaecology (2004) has published evidence-based guidelines as part of the procedures for establishing informed consent to abortion. They recommend that abortion providers tell women that only a small minority of women experience any long-term adverse psychological sequelae after an abortion.

A woman friendly mental health service

The Women's Health Council's report *Women's Mental Health: Promoting a Gendered Approach to Policy and Service Provision* is to be published in 2005. This will undoubtedly contribute to the debate about delivering a woman-centred mental health service. In the UK, a Department of Health report refers to research on views of women service users, survivors and carers who consistently state that, in addition to their fundamental right to 'be kept safe', they want:

• Services which will promote empowerment
• Choice and self-determination
• To place importance on the underlying causes and context of their distress in addition to their symptoms
• To address important issues relating to their role as mothers
• The needs for safe accommodation and access to education
• Training and work opportunities
• Value their strengths, abilities and potential for recovery (UK Department of Health, 2002: 9–10)

The UK report outlines the requirements for developing gender sensitive mental health care. They suggest that single sex services are essential in some cases. Other important factors to be taken into account include: the expressed preference of women to have choices available; the specific gender, cultural or religious needs of different groups of women; the creation of a safe environment which has particular relevance to women with experience of violence and abuse; the particular needs of women with sexually disinhibited behaviour, older women and lesbian women (2002: 10). There is a need to develop and strengthen specialist services in all of these areas.

Promoting Women's Health: A Population Investment for Ireland's Future was published by the Women's Health Council in 2002. It included proposals for achieving significant health gain for women. It demanded that the Department of Health and Children develop criteria, models, structures and procedures for the integration of gender considerations into national and regional practice related to the health of women. It led to the establishment of the National Planning Forum for Women's Health, which presented an interim report in 2003. This covered a range of topics central to women's health:

- The low visibility of women's health issues and of a gender dimension in general in health policy documents
- The need for gender responsive planning to deal with the gendered manifestation of health and disease
- The identification of a gender impact assessment mechanism as a tool for estimating the impact of policy and structural change
- The need for health data to be disaggregated by gender and age, disability and ethnicity to facilitate the development of performance indicators at national and regional levels
- The development of guidelines and a budget for gender mainstreaming
- A gender dimension should be added into health policy planning

The Forum indicated that women specific targets and actions are also necessary. It concluded that there is a commonality of disadvantage shared by all women as a result of gender, which is frequently manifested in sub-optimal health.

Conclusion

Mental health is just one aspect of a woman's biography and, as this chapter has shown, is very closely related to the strains of living as a woman in society today. These include gender stereotyping, multiple roles of being carer and breadwinner, lack of resources to cope with those roles and, for some women, the experience of living with intimate violence. These issues can be dealt with only by structural change within a wider social context. It is important to focus on the general position in which women find themselves in Irish society.

Ireland still remains a society in which the majority of women become mothers and this specific role for women is still enshrined in the Constitution. As there is a relationship between support and psychological well-being, access to comprehensive, affordable and responsive health and counselling services for all women is essential. Women's economic power, access to childcare, training, education and employment as well as security and safety are prerequisites for good mental health.

Chapter 9

Ageing and mental health

Mary Drury

Introduction

This chapter will begin with an historical exploration of the Irish response to the mental health needs of older people and will discuss current policy with particular reference to dementia and depression as both conditions are recognised as being the greatest mental health challenges faced by older people. The focus on dementia *per se* is valid since much of the recent literature and philosophy of dementia care have a resonance in respect of care approaches to other mental health conditions associated with ageing. A brief overview of a European perspective, in addition to the primary issues and challenges faced by health and social care systems as attitudinal shifts occur in the wider western world, will also be given. Finally the chapter will address how some of the issues should be comprehensively addressed to 'fit' with changing needs and expectations.

Little survives to tell us how ageing was viewed in classical antiquity. Galen (AD 130–200), physician to a school of gladiators, saw old age as 'the driest time of life'. His diagnosis is profoundly pessimistic, what after all is old age, other than 'the pathway to death'? Other writers and philosophers have testified in words that may say more about their personal anxieties than about the values of their culture: Cicero vaunted the wisdom that accompanies age, whereas the prospect of growing older filled Seneca with dread. By the medieval period, the virtue of a healthy old age contrasted with the symbolism of Christian art – a strange amalgam of signs of sagacity (white hair) and sin (withered skin). The Shakespearean image of the ages of man as 'steps' ascending from infancy to an adult podium followed by descent and decline emerges to form a persistent metaphor (Blaikie, 1999). Today, ageism is endemic in western societies (Blytheway, 2001) and influences all areas of economic and social policy (Townsend, 1986). For older Westerners who face challenges to their mental health, their ageing is further exacerbated by the stigma that attaches to conditions such as depression and dementia.

It has been generally acknowledged that there is no accepted age at which a person becomes *old*, and that our determination of old age in the western world has largely been defined in chronological terms with origins in bureaucratic necessity. However, defining ageing in chronological terms has largely contributed to the treatment of people over the age of 65 years as a homogeneous group, and as a consequence they have frequently been marginalised. The literature of recent years has emphasised the importance of understanding the variety of circumstances and experiences which constitutes older age (Walker, 1986, Fennell et al., 1988; Hugman, 1994). Such understanding is vital to correct what Hugman (1994) refers to as 'the "Monolithic" view of old age' which fails to take account of differences in gender, race ethnicity, disability or even age itself.

Gerontological research is now looking at future ageing cohorts in anticipation of the ageing of the 'baby boom' generation, which will significantly swell the proportion of older people in western countries by the year 2010. Researchers suggest that this group will have different values and lifestyles from those born before the Second World War, and that they will redefine the ageing experience just as they redefined adolescence and middle age (Silverstone, 2000). A range of constructs, theoretical models and practical concerns shapes concepts of mental health and mental illness in later life. Indeed the concept of mental health, as of physical health, goes beyond the absence of disease or disorder. Evidence about the preventive benefits of 'wellness' and 'successful ageing' have focused on the importance of defining mental health – even though the mental health delivery network in the western world is based on a medical model that addresses only illness and disorder (Honn Qualls, 2002). Implied is some subjective notion of 'well-being'. Research in the field of lifespan psychology indicates factors that constitute psychological well-being. Rowe and Kahn (1998) define successful ageing as the ability to maintain three key behaviours or characteristics:

- A low risk of disease and disease related disability
- High mental and physical functioning
- Active engagement with life

However, the construct of old age and mental illness as a biomedical problem remains dominant and has impacted enormously on policy making, and on the nature of service delivery and professional care.

A historical overview

Records from the time of the Brehon Laws show that there was within Ireland's kin system an obligation 'to care' for those who were aged, insane or suffering from a disability (O' Connor, 1995). There was no institution to address the specific needs of the mentally ill until 1745, when Jonathan Swift, Dean of St

Patrick's Cathedral, founded St Patrick's Hospital (Burke, 1987). In the early nineteenth century the mentally ill were the responsibility of the Lord Lieutenant's department, with the Richmond Asylum (later to be called St Brendan's Hospital) accepting 'lunatics' from all over Ireland. Gross over-crowding was the result, and the dreadful conditions at the facility led to the establishment in 1817 of District Lunatic Asylums. A change in how these asylums were managed came in 1862: operational control was passed from the 'Moral Governor', a layman, to the medical profession (Burke, 1987). The latter part of the nineteenth century saw an increasing awareness of the need for refinement of the Poor Law, and with it an overhaul of the workhouse system. The Commissions on Poor Law Reform of 1903 and 1909 recommended that the elderly and infirm should be placed in separate institutions. However, the recommendation was not acted upon, and the Poor Law Relief Commission of 1927 proposed that the former workhouses, later to be known as 'County Homes', accommodate both the elderly and infirm.

The bias towards institutional care remained strong until the emergence of documents such as *The Care of the Aged Report* (Inter-Departmental Committee, 1968) and *The Years Ahead: A Policy for the Elderly* (Department of Health, 1988). In Irish terms, *The Years Ahead* was a breakthrough because, for the first time at policy level, the old, negative, 'workhouse' attitude to illness in the elderly was discarded; and a more subtle approach, which we would recognise as 'modern', adopted in its stead (Clinch, 1998). This shift in emphasis became more pronounced in subsequent reports and culminated in the setting of a target within the strategy for effective health care entitled *Shaping a Healthier Future* (Department of Health, 1994b) to ensure that 90 per cent of people over 75 years continued to live at home.

Advocates of change repeatedly emphasised the importance of introducing new structures and facilities with appropriate statutory funding to cope with the impending demographic changes, and of supporting policy with a legislative infrastructure. *The Years Ahead* (1988) was adopted as official policy by the Department of Health and served as a blueprint for service planning and development at that time. However, its real impetus was lost because its publication coincided with a downturn in the economy; the legislation necessary for its support was not enacted and it underestimated the growth in numbers of the population aged over 75 years.

Mental health policy and planning

A study group was appointed in 1981 to review the psychiatric services and its report, *The Psychiatric Services: Planning for the Future* (Department of Health, 1984), was published in 1984. The psychiatric hospital was the focal point of service delivery to those with mental health difficulties. The elderly were among the report's primary concerns, and the prevention of psychiatric illness at a primary care level was a fundamental recommendation. Also addressed in *The Psychiatric Services: Planning for the Future* was the need to determine the division of responsibility between psychiatric and geriatric services for the 'elderly mentally infirm'. This was particularly emphasised in the context of dementia, and the report advised that the majority of those with a dementia 'should be cared for by the primary care or geriatric service' (Department of Health, 1984: 89). It was also suggested that the medical needs of the majority of those with a dementia could be met by the primary care services or by the geriatric services, with psychiatry to provide appropriate support. The report proposed the appointment of old age psychiatrists to provide specialist assessment and treatment services for older people with mental health problems. One of the more positive health developments in Ireland over the last ten years has been the appointment of old age psychiatrists to most of the country's health boards.

   The Psychiatric Services: Planning for the Future (Department of Health, 1984) reiterated the official policy line that treatment services for the elderly should ensure they remain in their own homes for as long as possible. The report also envisaged that this could be achieved by developing a comprehensive preventative programme that would prepare people for old age and help them to retain their independence. In 1992, a Green Paper on Mental Health (Department of Health, 1992) was published to review progress in the development of a new psychiatric service following the recommendations of *The Psychiatric Services: Planning for the Future* (Department of Health, 1984). This paper also explored the new legislation needed to replace the Mental Treatment Act of 1945. It was followed by a White Paper in 1995 entitled *A New Mental Health Act* (Department of Health, 1995b). One of its proposals was to expand the definition of 'mental disorder' to include 'severe dementia' (1995: 20–1) which is sometimes associated with severe behavioural disturbance. The new Mental Health Act, introduced in 2001, took account of guidelines and principles enshrined in a range of international conventions. The Mental Health Commission, which was established in 2002, is the vehicle to ensure implementation of the provisions of the Act. The fundamental objective of the Commission is the promotion of quality in the delivery of services and a key priority is the development and enhancement of relationships with the stakeholders.

   The publication of *An Action Plan on Dementia* (O'Shea and O'Reilly, 1999) was welcomed as a major milestone. It was the first time that the issue of dementia was analysed in terms of resource implications, existing policy, the balance of care issues and the different pathways to care. The guiding principle of this report was the recognition of the individuality of the person with dementia and of his or her needs.

The comprehensive nature of the report, the methodology it employed of consultation with a range of national organisations, including professionals and advocacy groups, and the resultant recommendations, provide a blueprint for future policy and planning. 'The overall goal of the plan is to describe a best practice model for dementia care in Ireland' (O'Shea and O'Reilly, 1999: 26). The Health Strategy Document of 2001 included a commitment to establishing 'a clear framework for implementation of the recommendations contained in reports on health promotion and dementia' (Department of Health and Children, 2001b: 149).

In 1998, the Department of Health and Children established the Dementia Services Information and Development Centre. The remit of the Centre is to serve as a resource for professionals, formal caregivers, service providers and health administrators working in the field of dementia care. It was born of a debate in the early nineties about Ireland's preparedness to respond appropriately to the needs of people with dementia. The Centre's main activities include the dissemination of information on all aspects of dementia, the provision of education and training, and the development of specialised research within Ireland and of research partnerships with others in Europe, United States and Australia. These dementia-related initiatives have demonstrated the beginnings of a shift from a philosophy of care dominated by the bio-medical model (Convery, 1998), with all of its attendant nihilism and stigma, to a philosophy of care driven by a definition of dementia as a form of disability. Kitwood (1997) illustrated the critical differences between the two cultures of care created by the bio-medical and disability models. He stated that the person's experience of their condition was largely dependent on the quality of care they were offered. This approach to dementia has a growing influence on current thinking in most of the western world, and as a result has created a change in how care is conceptualised (Stokes and Goudie, 1990; Goldsmith, 1996; Kitwood, 1997; Cheston and Bender, 1999).

A European perspective

Most European countries promote policies for 'ageing in place' that form the basis of 'community care' programmes. Interest in older people in the European Union (EU) burgeoned in the early 1990s with the establishment of the Commission's Observatory on Ageing and Older People, the first programme for older people initiated in 1991 (Tester, 1996). Changing forms of service provision and levels of finance impact on people who need care and, because of the heterogeneity of the population, change affects people differently. These effects transcend national borders. Policies may be informed by 'borrowing' or 'learning' from other countries with similar political priorities, and socio-economic or demographic profiles. Hence collaborative research partnerships and alliances, many funded by the EU, have led to a cross fertilisation of ideas and a sharing of experiences.

One such study, *The European Trans-national Alzheimer's Study* (ETAS), (Warner et al., 1998) documented the findings of investigations that were carried out on both the general national health and the social care policies across 15 European member states. The study also investigated more specific policies in relation to old age care, dementia care, and support. A review of policy in member states highlighted substantial agreement on key principles of policy. The driving force behind this convergence was deemed to be twofold:

Politio-economic

With the rapidly growing demands of older people as a result of their increasing numbers, the growth in the numbers of those with a dementia, and the financial and political implications of failing to provide the most cost-effective state and allied supports for them, the member states share a similar future demographic pattern of increasing numbers of elderly and very elderly citizens and a decline in the proportion of citizens of working age.

Humanitarian

General recognition also emerged from Warner et al.'s (1998) study that the quality of the support provided in the past was no longer acceptable. Key developments in this area have been professionally led, as with the Health Advisory Service reports in the UK. They have also been led by bodies more closely allied to national political structures such as the National Council on Ageing and Older People in Ireland, which serves as the advisory body to the Minister for Health and Children. These developments have been complemented by the growth of patients' and carers' advocacy and support groups such as the Alzheimer's Society and Mental Health Ireland and an increased articulation of the values and priorities of older people in general. The ETAS Report (Warner et al., 1998) suggested that developments in dementia-related policies reflect the development of broader health and social welfare policies for older people. In many European countries, congruence has materialised as two previously distinct streams have merged – the framework developed for people with a mental illness (with an emphasis on the protection of those unable to safeguard their own affairs) and policies on the general older person in which the focus has on been the maintenance of independence.

The primary issues

The population of Ireland is ageing, and it is anticipated that the number of people aged over 65 years in the year 2011 will be in the region of 521,700. Of greater significance is the expected increase in the numbers of older old people, that is, those over 80 years: it is among this group that the prevalence of dementia is highest (Jorm et al., 1987). These projected increases in the older population, coupled with an increased prevalence of mental health problems, have enormous implications for the health and social care services.

The Psychiatric Services: Planning for the Future (Department of Health, 1984), made a distinction between three groups of older people with mental health difficulties.

1   Older people with functional mental illness, that is those over 65 years who develop a difficulty such as depression for the first time or who experience a relapse
2   Older people with a dementia
3   Older people with a long-standing psychiatric problem such as a bi-polar disorder

Using a framework 'the pathway to psychiatric care', described by Goldberg and Huxley (1980, 1992), it has been suggested that 26–31 per cent of the adult population in any one year will live in the community with a mental disorder. Within that framework, dementia and depression represent the two most serious challenges to mental health faced by people as they age. While such conditions also occur in the young, it has been well established that dementia is predominantly a disorder of older adults with its incidence and prevalence increasing with age (Ritchie and Kildea, 1995). Approximately five per cent of people over 65 have a dementia, and the figure increases to 20 per cent of those aged over 80.

Dementia is an umbrella term used to describe a range of conditions and syndromes. The most common form is Alzheimer's disease that accounts for approximately 50 per cent of all dementias. Marshall (1998) defines dementia as a disability, characterised by impairments in memory, in reasoning, in the ability to engage in new learning; it is associated with a high level of stress and with an acute sensitivity to the social and built environment.

Depression is an emotional state characterised by feelings of hopelessness and sadness and when such feelings become prolonged or are disproportionate to the personal circumstances of the individual, they may be deemed to need intervention. Depression is also a common late-life mental disorder entailing considerable disability, and, as many epidemiological studies bear out, is deserving of attention and full intervention in its own right (Kirby, 2003).

Blazer et al. (1991) found that an association between age and depressive symptoms was positive and statistically significant. Other factors too, such as chronic illness, cognitive impairment, and a lack of social support, influence the development of depressive symptoms (Kennedy et al., 1989; O'Hara et al., 1985). This association was mirrored in the prevalence study of mental disorders in older people carried out in Dublin, among community-dwelling elderly (Lawlor et al., 1994). This study found that 13.1 per cent of those aged over 65 in an urban community had a diagnosable depression. The study further showed that 9.7 per cent of older people could be classified as having sub-cases of depression, that is, a variety of depressive symptoms.

Data from international studies reveal similar rates of depression for community dwellers with approximately 14–18 per cent of those who attend their general practitioner doing so with depressive symptoms (Keogh and Roche, 1996; Denihan et al., 2000). Some studies have found that depression among the community-dwelling elderly is under-diagnosed and under-treated by general practitioners, while Goldberg and Huxley (1980) estimated that as many as 50 per cent of cases of mild or moderate depression are missed by general practitioners. It has been suggested that factors such as medical illness, bereavement and somatisation (i.e. presentation of physical complaints as depression) make diagnosis difficult (Lawlor, 1995).

Suicide rates in most industrialised nations increase with age (Vaillant and Blumenthal, 1990; Diekstra, 1993). In almost all countries the highest rate is found amongst males aged 75 years and over (Keogh and Roche, 1996). Suicidal behaviour in older people is undertaken with greater intent and with greater lethality than in younger age groups. Depressive illness is the most common predictor of suicide among older people, but social factors and medical illness are also highlighted in the literature. Although an established dementia is likely to be a protective factor, the significance of an early dementia is a matter of speculation that has received scant attention. For some individuals, the fear of dependency and of ending life in an 'institution' is an important dynamic, irrespective of the presence of cognitive deficits (Cattell, 2000). The Irish Association of Suicidology in the Proceedings of the Eighth Annual Conference (2004), entitled 'Suicide and Older People' suggests that one in ten Irish suicides is among older people, and again the issue of under-diagnosis and under-treatment of depression was highlighted.

A further obstacle to the accurate diagnosis of depression in older people is that depression can mimic some of the symptoms of dementia and may also co-occur with dementia. The ability to identify, follow up and intervene earlier would require considerable development of existing services, with more advanced liaison services between old age psychiatry and medicine for older people, and greater availability of memory clinics (Kirby, 2003).

Depression, dementia and the care continuum

In view of the fact that both depression and dementia are to the fore as mental health difficulties to be faced by many older people, it is useful here to analyse some of the key components of the care continuum. These include the assessment and diagnostic process, community-based services and supports, and residential care. The diagnosis and management of mental health difficulties are facilitated by a thorough assessment, usually undertaken by a general practitioner. For some older people, however, these initial steps may be difficult, as there may be significant variations in general practitioner responses to the issues, needs and concerns of older people. The use of appropriate assessment scales and tools may also be problematic for some general practitioners. Others may not be comfortable dealing with social, cognitive and behavioural problems and may be reluctant to label someone as having a dementia because of the negativity and stigma associated with the diagnosis (O'Shea and O'Reilly, 1999).

General practitioners need to have knowledge of the assessment process, knowledge about dementia itself, an awareness of carer stress, a route to sources of help, and knowledge of the reasons for seeking specialist assessment (Iliffe, 1994). The availability of new drug therapies to slow the progression of the disease process has added weight to the importance of an early and accurate diagnosis. The benefits are considerable in that cognitive impairment arising from a simple deficiency such as Vitamin B12 can be established and treated, depression may be diagnosed and treated, and, if a dementia is confirmed, the person with dementia and their family may be linked with the appropriate supports. Brodaty (1988) suggests that early diagnosis also affords the opportunity to inform the person of the nature of their condition as well as facilitating family decision-making and planning for future care. This would, for example, include the provision of an Enduring Power of Attorney to facilitate the management of finances.

It is important to acknowledge that people with dementia may comprise a relatively small percentage of a general practitioner's practice list (Eccles et al., 1998). Nevertheless, given the excess disability that results from inappropriate care, and the growing therapeutic optimism in dementia care, there is a compelling need to improve the primary care response (Downs, 2000).

Referral to a consultant geriatrician or psycho-geriatrician may occur, either to seek a differential diagnosis to determine the type of dementia or because the person concerned is exhibiting behavioural problems. Access to a 'memory clinic' to seek a differential diagnosis of dementia and to address co-morbidity or otherwise of a depression is at present inequitable. Memory clinics are an alternative service model: they offer close liaison between old age psychiatry and medicine for older people and have a proven track record (Swanwick et al.,

1996). While there are now a number of such clinics within the Eastern Regional Health Authority area, other health board areas are less well served.

The public health nurse is a key player at primary care level and in that capacity has a critical role in identifying older people with mental health difficulties. Given the 'cradle to grave' nature of this service, with the attendant time constraints, the range of client/patient needs and a concomitant expectation of a high level of expertise, it may be timely to suggest the division of this service to establish a specialism dedicated to the needs of older people. Screening for depression and for dementia needs to be proactive and community-based. Home assessments by various disciplines working with older people have been endorsed as a sign of good practice (Audit Commission, 2002) and have been recommended as the first stage of care management (Richardson and Orrell, 2002). The need to have a dedicated community-based social work service to meet the needs of older people has long been highlighted in Irish reports, including the *Action Plan for Dementia* (O'Shea and O'Reilly, 1999). This initiative has been slow to develop, yet a small number of appointments have been made and it is expected that this service will continue to grow.

Who cares? Community care or family care?

The answer to these questions will not come from solving an equation that balances the family with the hospital. Caring for older people is a complex multidisciplinary task (Horton, 1997). Unfortunately, the usual pattern of progression of dementia means that people need considerable care, often for several years. Much of this care is undertaken in domestic settings, some in residential settings (Mc Namee et al., 1999). Care for people with dementia, whatever the setting, can strain the resources of individuals, families, communities and potentially healthcare systems (Burns et al., 2001).

While Irish families, like their European counterparts, continue to be the main providers of care of older relatives, this caring potential is decreasing because of changing family structures. Smaller families, women in paid employment, greater mobility, and relationship breakdown will likely contribute to a reduction in the numbers of available family carers (Daatland, 1996; Swanwick and Lawlor, 1998). When a wide range of European citizens was asked whether families were now less willing to look after elderly relatives, the overwhelming reply was 'Yes' (Walker and Maltby, 1997). A care gap is deepening and few countries are addressing this pressing concern (Horton, 1997).

The difficulties associated with Ireland's community care infrastructure have been well documented in literature and in many reports, including the *Review of the Years Ahead* (Ruddle et al., 1997) and *An Action Plan on Dementia* (O'Shea and O'Reilly, 1999). Legislation is essential to ensure standards of care

(Ruddle et al., 1997) and the piecemeal, ad hoc nature of vital services such as the home help service and twilight services has left them prey to changes in economic fortunes, with a consequent impact on those who require their input. The failure to enshrine recommendations in statutory form ultimately means that there is no obligation on the part of health boards to provide community care services (Fitzgerald, 2000). Overall there is a lack of continuity and an unco-ordinated delivery of services from agencies, which frequently operate independently of one another. There is inequity and inefficiency and an ideology that seems intent on the separation of health and social care. The failure to legislate a community care act is in marked contrast to the fact that legislation has been enacted in relation to nursing care, the Health (Nursing Homes) Act 1990. When this is viewed against the target set within the strategy for effective health care entitled *Shaping a Healthier Future* (Department of Health, 1994b) that 90 per cent of people aged 75 plus should live in their own homes, a significant credibility gap is apparent.

Residential care

Many older people with mental health difficulties will need to take up residential care. The literature has recognised that the residential care needs of people with dementia are quite different and the trend in other countries is to provide care in specialist dementia care settings, frequently attached to more mainstream residential facilities. This trend is in its infancy in Ireland. There is international consensus on what constitutes 'good design' of such an environment (Judd et al., 1998; Calkins, 1988) and some measure of expert agreement on the characteristics of a specialist unit:

- Admission of residents with cognitive impairment
- Specialist trained staff
- Appropriate activity programming
- Active family involvement
- A segregated and modified physical and social environment
                                        (Mentes and Buckwalter, 1998).

Since its inception, one of the tasks undertaken by the Dementia Services Information and Development Centre has been the dissemination of information on best practice in designing or modifying dementia care environments. In addition, research on Irish day centre and residential care environments has been undertaken (Cahill et al., 2003). The majority of people with dementia who are in residential care are living in generic facilities. While there are no statistics available in relation to the numbers of residents with mental health problems such as dementia, it has been suggested that between one third and one half of all residents have a dementia (Ineichen, 1990). One of the recommendations made in the report on *Mental Disorders in Older Irish People* (Keogh and Roche, 1996) was that future audits of residential care settings should provide more detailed information on the medical and psychosocial status of residents. Appropriately detailed information sought at the time of admission would go some way towards redressing this difficulty.

The way forward

The challenges for the future in relation to mental health and ageing can be set broadly within a framework utilised by Ruddle (1998), which incorporated six key actions.

1 Developing a vision of ageing and older life
The term 'active ageing' was adopted by the World Health Organisation in the late 1990s, to convey a more inclusive message than 'healthy ageing' and to recognise the factors in addition to health care that affect how individuals and populations age (Kalache and Kickbusch, 1997). The active ageing approach is based on the recognition of the human rights of older people and the United Nations' Principles of Independence, participation, dignity, care and self-fulfilment. It shifts strategic planning away from a needs-based approach (which assumes that older people are passive targets) to a rights-based approach that recognises the rights of people to equality of opportunity and treatment in all aspects of life as they grow older. It supports their responsibility to exercise their participation in the political process and other aspects of community life. The Equality Authority report, *Implementing Equality for Older People* (2002), has set an agenda for change which should help to counteract negative perspectives of a person's age and capacities, respect diversity and ensure the right of older people to participate and have equality of outcomes.

Health promotion tends to have as its focus physical health and the population in general. The mental health needs of older people require particular emphasis to include preparation for retirement, education about social issues such as housing, and legal matters and education about issues such as dealing with loss and bereavement and maintenance of social contact. The identification of specific tangible areas where improvements in the health and well-being of older people could be enhanced was cited as one of the challenges in a report entitled *Adding Years to Life and Life to Years: A Health Promotion Strategy For Older People* (Brenner and Shelley, 1998). Future health promotion programmes should take account of the strong links that exist between psychological well-being and physical health status (Fahey and Murray, 1994). The focus should therefore include psychological preparation for ageing and its associated changes in addition to the prevention of illness (Keogh and Roche, 1996).

2   Including the consumer in planning and service development

There is a growing awareness of the need to include the voice of the older person in all areas of planning and service development. In the case of dementia this fits with current thinking and best practice in a number of areas. These include: hearing the voice of the person with dementia at the broadest level (Goldsmith, 1996); sharing the diagnosis with the person; planning for their future and eventually perhaps realising advanced directives in relation to care issues and outcomes. (Goldsmith, 1996; Barnett, 2000; Killick and Allan, 2001). Barnett (1997: 1), in evaluating a service for people with dementia that included users' perceptions of services, described how people are 'sidelined from the collaborative process which potentially exists between service agencies and family carers'. The Irish Dementia Services Information and Development Centre is currently working on research to elicit the subjective experiences of people with dementia who attended a memory clinic for diagnosis.

Older people are not a homogeneous group and their increasing numbers should not be viewed as a burden on society. Older people have a right to full citizenship which includes the right to have one's voice heard at the decision-making level, thus one of the recommendations of the National Council on Ageing and older People is that 'older people should have recognition in their own right in the Social Partnership process' (Garavan et al., 2001: 58). Unless the voice of the older person is actively included, they will continue to be the objects of political, medical and economic discourse rather than subjects voicing their own concerns (Blaikie, 1999: 3).

3   Adopting a holistic approach to need

The fusion of medical and social care approaches is vital, with a view to recognising mental health difficulties as conditions that disable some aspects of an individual's ability to function. Case management has been identified in a US Congress Report (Office of Technology Assessment, 1990) as being one of four elements necessary to ensure an effective system to link older people to their required services; the other components are public education, information, and referral and outreach. The National Council on Ageing and Older People has also recommended the introduction of care management as a means of health and social care delivery in a number of its reports (Browne, 1992; Ruddle et al., 1997; O'Shea and O'Reilly, 1999; Delaney et al., 2001; Garavan et al., 2001). This is a system for the planning, co-ordination and delivery of tailor made services for vulnerable older people at local level which is achieved through consultation with the older person, their carer(s) and the local health and social services professionals. Conditions such as depression and dementia demand a bio-psycho-social approach and therefore there is a need to provide for comprehensive needs assessment with community-based teams for older people. The Lewisham Case Management scheme was established in the

United Kingdom to provide care management in a community-based service for mental health of older people. The implications of the approach to mental health diagnosis, treatment and the operation of the team are discussed in a number of papers (MacDonald et al., 1994, Von Abendorff et al., 1994; Brown et al., 1995; Challis et al., 1997). Approximately 20–25 per cent of those aged 65 years will be affected by a mental health difficulty at any one time (Lawlor et al., 1994) with an attendant ripple effect on other family members, in addition to the likelihood that the older person may also have a physical health problem. Given these facts, the rationale for a case management approach to the older person in the community is strong.

4 Providing options within a continuum of care
Fundamental to the provision of a continuum of care is the need to have a legislative framework: a community care act. There is no shortage of imaginative policy ideas to frame that legislation in the recommendations of reports such as *An Action Plan on Dementia* (O'Shea and O'Reilly, 1999) and *Mental Disorders in Older Irish People: Incidence and Prevalence and Treatment* (Keogh and Roche, 1996). As older people are not a homogeneous group, neither also are those with different mental health difficulties. A range of service options should therefore be available which can be tailored to individual need and fit with best practice in the respective fields. Ireland's response to the mental health needs of its older people demands new service configurations and a commitment to a holistic approach involving assessment and understanding of the person's routine. Challis (2000) has also recommended intervention at a pace and in ways that are acceptable to the older person, the involvement and support of family members in care plans and risk assessment and minimisation through anticipation and planning. Challis (2000) also stresses the importance of having the resources and infrastructure to meet the needs of clients.

5 Evaluating outcomes and research solutions
Quality outcome measures reflecting health and social need should be established and should reflect best practice in standards of care. Agencies that promote research and service development need to be appropriately funded, and collaboration should be encouraged that is representative of consumers, advocacy groups, and public/private and statutory/voluntary alliances or partnerships. Measurement of quality of life (QoL) has become a major feature of much social and epidemiological research in health and social care settings, and has been widely undertaken by collaborative partnerships within the European Union. Higgs et al. (2003) argue that the thrust of this work has focused on measures of health and illness as equivalents of QoL, and that this response has been reductionist as old age is viewed as a dimension of health, disability and disease. The model espoused by the authors is derived from

aspects of social theory and is based on needs-satisfaction within four domains, control, autonomy, pleasure and self-realisation. Their model reflected a model of healthy ageing discussed in an earlier study by Bryant et al. (2001), which examined older people's determination of what constituted healthy ageing. The reframing of healthy ageing in older people's own terms promotes the need for interdisciplinary support of their desired goals and outcomes rather than medical approaches to deficits and challenges.

6 Providing for intersectoral input and involvement of the consumer

In the context of mental health, such provision recognises the many players involved in responding to the range of difficulties being experienced; and the need to facilitate the education of older people themselves, their families, and the professionals and formal caregivers who are involved with them. Regional and local-level partnerships are desirable that include health services, housing authorities, social welfare and voluntary organisations, with the older person, where feasible, an equal partner. The proposal by the Department of Health and Children to set up an expert group, which would undertake the task of preparing a national policy framework for the development of mental health services, will be a step to ensuring all voices are heard including that of the service user. Ireland is no longer a monoculture and thus one of the challenges to be faced in mental health is to recognise the impact of cultural values on ageing and, by implication, the nature of cultural diversity on issues such as dementia and depression.

In conclusion, if care is considered primarily as an 'economic problem', the cultural and ethical values of a society will be compromised (Cohen, et al., 1997). As Blaikie puts it:

> [Today] people remain fitter for longer, and morbidity is compressed into an abbreviated final phase. Such a transformation reflects a major health achievement, yet we appear to be ill equipped to address the social, personal and political needs that it creates. Ageing societies have in fact become victims of their own success. However, attitudes have shifted less than the social realities behind them, perhaps because older people have been objects of discourse, more than they have been citizens speaking in their own right. Sadly, if anything has remained a constant it has been the perception of older people as elderly others, rather than the embodiment of our future selves. (Blaikie, 1999: iv, 3)

Chapter 10

Dual diagnosis in mental health

Michael Timms

Introduction

Traditionally, a person with a learning disability who uses mental health services is described as someone with a 'dual diagnosis'. This alliterative label can be confusing when not given a context as it could refer to the person described above or to a person with addiction problems who also has a mental health difficulty. The latter is often the case in the US (see, for example, Dual Diagnosis Recovery Network, 1996). Beguilingly, 'dual diagnosis' suggests a discrete category of people, a neat grouping that can be herded, sectioned, and then treated or serviced. However, we do know that people have multiple identities: a person with mobility impairment in the Traveller community who is a woman cannot adequately be described as a person with a disability. Such a term leaves out, or excludes, so much of her identity, not to mention the issues she faces in modern Irish society. We need descriptors for people which capture the richness of their identity. A lengthy label like 'people with learning disabilities who use mental health services' may not be entirely satisfactory, but it does avoid the 'flat pack' approach of service management shorthand. More importantly, it is also the term that many service users prefer to see applied to themselves. Therefore, in this chapter the term 'dual diagnosis' will be taken to refer to those with a learning disability who also have mental health difficulties.

Identifying those with dual diagnosis

The accurate measurement of the population who have a learning disability on its own is somewhat problematic. The questions on disability which were put in the 2002 Census of Population do not appear to permit an assessment of the incidence of learning disability in the community, and that may not have been the intention. It is not within the remit of this chapter to reflect on the implications of the absence of such data for the planning of government expenditure. Instead, focus will be on which demographic data of the disabled population are available, provided primarily by the databases created by health service professionals.

The National Intellectual Disability Database was established during 1995 with the stated aims:

1 To improve the accuracy of data available to health boards on the population of people with an intellectual disability
2 To enable the current needs of people with an intellectual disability to be assessed more accurately
3 To support planning for the future development of services for people with an intellectual disability

It also aspires to 'facilitate . . . the generation of a national census' (HRB, 1997: 1).

The first aim above suggests a broad sweep of the canvas, which might indeed facilitate the generation of a national census. However, the reality is contained in the third aim that refers to 'planning' or 'development of services'. The figures collected in the first Annual Report of the Database Committee include almost all persons 'with a moderate, severe or profound intellectual disability' (HRB, 1997: 2) precisely because such people are current and continuing users of services. These are individuals who are easily captured by any recording system that works through services, as this database does. The report goes on to state that for many reasons it was not considered desirable to register all persons with a mild intellectual disability (1997: 2). The reasons for this omission are not specified by the authors, but may include the fact that because many of these people do not use services of any kind, they therefore cannot be recorded by the database. In short, the database – with its focus on services – does not give us a clear picture of the learning disabled population. This points to the clear need for appropriate questions in the national census.

Greater difficulties exist in assessing the numbers of those with a learning disability who also have a mental health difficulty from the information available in the database. The Annual Report of the National Intellectual Disability Database Committee 2002 does provide figures of the number of people with a learning difficulty in psychiatric hospitals ($N = 515$) and the number in 'Intensive Placement – Challenging Behaviour' settings ($N = 284$) (HRB, 2003: 34) because these are residential placements. The majority of those recorded on the database are only in receipt of some kind of day service, and the day service data do not capture so precisely the reason why these people are in a particular service. This results in a lack of information on the range of mental health difficulties in this population from the database.

The National Psychiatric In-Patient Reporting System also yields limited information on those with dual diagnosis. The most recent report available (Daly and Walsh, 2001) states that the diagnosis returned for 275 people admitted to psychiatric hospitals in 2000 was 'Mental Handicap'. Such information does not allow for an understanding of the mental health needs of people who have learning difficulties and who find themselves in hospital. Some at least may be there for historical reasons that have little to do with mental health and more to do with lack of appropriate residential facilities. The National Psychiatric In-Patient Reporting System also highlights some of the labyrinthine recording systems still in existence in some psychiatric settings: 'Some hospitals do not diagnose until discharge, with the result that diagnosis is not available for any admission not discharged within the same year as admitted' (Daly and Walsh, 2001: 5).

The one piece of hard data that is to hand indicates that while 'the proportion of mentally handicapped persons in psychiatric hospitals has decreased in recent years, this still accounts for 10% of persons resident in hospital at the end of 2000' (Daly and Walsh, 2001: 3). This state of affairs where people with learning disabilities are inappropriately accommodated in Irish psychiatric hospitals has rightly drawn international criticism from both the UN Committee on Economic, Social and Cultural Rights (United Nations, 2002) and Amnesty International, the worldwide human rights organisation (Amnesty International, 2003).

Issues for people with learning difficulties who use mental health services

Despite the limited statistical data available on the population with dual diagnosis, it is important to explore policy issues for this group. The problems confronted by people with learning difficulties who use, or are required to use, mental health services are no different from those of any other section of Irish society making use of such services. They involve ensuring:

1   Informed consent to any treatment
2   Access to the full range of treatment options

The realisation of these goals is at the heart of what the US Standard Rules on the Equalisation of Opportunities for Persons with Disabilities (United Nations, 1994) has to say about the role of medical care as a pre-condition for equal opportunities. These two essentials for people with learning difficulties need to be considered and in so doing matters of concern to the wider population may also emerge.

Informed consent to treatment
Informed consent, or rather the lack of it, has bedevilled many aspects of Irish social history. Revelations on the way in which the state provided care services

to children of families deemed to be 'in need' have revealed gaps in understanding between what was on offer and what was actually delivered (Raftery and O'Sullivan, 1999). The consequences of such gaps were made painfully evident by Raftery's subsequent television documentary. Similar tales are told in relation to people with learning disabilities. Iacono and Murray (2003) quote a research study from the United States carried out at a residential institution for people with learning disabilities some decades ago. For the study, children were injected with hepatitis so that the natural history of the disease could be observed. Consent for the study rested solely with the management of the institution, and it is hard to see that either parents or children could have had an inkling of what was going on. Such a tale may seem to be the stuff of history, until attention is drawn to current press reports. The *New York Times* of 1 September 2003 reported several current federal investigations of institutions where children with disabilities were supposed to be receiving treatment:

> investigators from the civil rights division of the Justice Department recently found 'significant and wide-ranging deficiencies in patient care' at (institution identified). The hospital provides patients ages 11 to 17 with 'woefully inadequate' treatment and unnecessary medications, exposing them 'to a significant risk of harm and to actual harm' the Department said (Pear, 2003).

For people who use mental health services, the issue of consent to treatment was addressed in the Irish Mental Health Act 2001. Here consent is defined as:

> consent obtained freely without threats or inducements, where:
> a   The consultant psychiatrist responsible for the care and treatment of the patient is satisfied that the patient is capable of understanding the nature, purpose and likely effects of the proposed treatment; and
> b   The consultant psychiatrist has given the patient adequate information, in a form and language that the patient can understand, on the nature, purpose and likely effects of the proposed treatment. (Department of Health and Children, 2001d, Section 56)

This definition is laudable as far as it goes. But how does the psychiatrist decide, for example, on the 'form and language that the patient can understand' when he is meeting a distressed person with a learning disability for the first time. The Mental Health Act (Department of Health and Children 2001d) seems to suggest a way around such a dilemma:

> The consent of a patient shall be required for treatment except where, in the opinion of the consultant psychiatrist responsible for the care and treatment of the patient, the treatment is necessary to safeguard the life of the patient, to

restore his or her health, to alleviate his or her condition, or to relieve his or her suffering, and by reason of his or her mental disorder the patient is incapable of giving such consent. (Department of Health and Children, 2001d, Section 57)

Of concern here is the transparency of judgements and decisions a doctor has to make about 'risk to life', 'level of suffering' or the 'mental disorders' that seem to render a patient capable or incapable of giving consent. This is particularly important when the individual in question has a learning disability and requires from the psychiatrist a clear understanding of the nature of learning disability and the most effective way to communicate fully with that individual so that he/she is able make an informed choice about treatment.

'Consent by proxy' may be seen as a seemingly attractive alternative to use with people with a learning disability. Where individuals cannot give informed consent, a guardian or person/organisation having guardianship in law will give the consent. This is a system in use in Australia (National Health and Medical Research Council, 1999). However, there is a paucity of research on how surrogates (people who give consent by proxy) make their decision. One study, carried out in relation to medical research on older people, reported 46 per cent of surrogates refusing to give consent. Worryingly, the study also noted that 17 per cent of those who did give consent indicated their belief that the person for whom they spoke would not give consent if asked to do so (Warren et al., 1986). There is a further concern here. Many people with dual diagnosis are resident in 'generic intellectual disability centres' rather than in approved psychiatric facilities. Professionals involved in their care in these locations are not protected under the provisions of any of the mental health legislation. This is a serious concern, well understood by the professionals themselves, and about which they have clearly expressed their anxieties (NDA, 2003).

Access to the full range of treatment options

It is arguable that many marginalised groups and communities in Irish society are left on the sidelines with nothing that resembles an effective service. Those groups for whom we do make some sort of investment are presented with 'special' services. These are often delivered at sites remote from the mainstream community, a process that enhances marginalisation rather than combats it. The requirement to include people with disabilities by mainstreaming all services is the driving force behind *A Strategy for Equality*, the government report which is a blueprint for specific and appropriate action for those with disability (Commission on the Status of People with Disabilities, 1996).

Sadly, the view of inclusion and equity for persons with disability articulated in *A Strategy for Equality* has, in the main, failed to become a reality in policy terms. In 1996, the Department of Health published a discussion document containing clear proposals for the development of services to the learning disability sector (Department of Health, 1996). However, those proposals have never been implemented and the needs of those with learning disability have not been referred to in the more recent National Health Strategy (Department of Health and Children, 2001b).

Since the publication of the 2001 Health Strategy, a further review of the disability sector has appeared. This review included a survey across all health boards and relevant voluntary bodies, and the findings are almost predictable including

- The lack of a national service strategy for this client group
- An absence of joint planning by the Department of Health and Children across mental health and intellectual disability
- Mental health services are largely non-existent for persons living in the community either with family carers or independently
- An assumption that the mental health needs of this population are provided by the 'generic intellectual disability services' (NDA, 2003: 48–50)

The review goes on to recommend a service delivery model of which the cornerstone would be multi-disciplinary community-based mental health teams dedicated to this group of people. The staff on these teams would work as a specialist section of existing Community Area Mental Health Services and would be fully integrated with colleagues in the generic mental health service (NDA, 2003: 55–8). Challenges for the implementation of this model include finding a modus operandi for such multi-disciplinary teams within the current legislative framework which vests ultimate responsibility (and therefore control) in the hands of the medical profession; and the actual integration of these teams within the wider generic mental health service.

The former challenge is the greater. At a time when a number of physicians (Lynch, 2001), nursing and paramedical staff (Barker et al., 1998), and service users (Faulkner, 2000) are questioning both the validity and the efficacy of medical interventions for mental health difficulties, it is vital that services make available the full range of therapeutic interventions. People with learning disabilities who need to use mental health services can make use of diagnostic instruments like the Beck Depression Inventory (Rusiecki and Alfinito, 1997) and the dexamethasone suppression test (Vitiello and Behar, 1992) with the same validity as any other patient. More crucially, there is also evidence that this group of people respond well to the gentler therapies, including psycho-dynamic (Berry, 2003) and psychoanalytic (De Groef and Heinemann, 1999) approaches.

While gentler techniques for the treatment of mental illness for those with learning disability seem indicated, it is unlikely that these therapies, and others like them, will become available through medically led, multi-disciplinary teams. This gives cause for concern when questions are currently being posed about both the safety and the effectiveness of some drug-based medical interventions. For instance, the usefulness of anti-psychotic drugs in controlling challenging behaviour has been addressed in a large number of studies. Brylewski and Duggan (1999) assessed over 500 of these and found only three that were methodologically sound, randomised controlled trials. None of the three was able to show whether antipsychotic drugs were beneficial or not in controlling challenging behaviour. Ashcroft et al. (2001) have cautioned that the benefit of these drugs for those with challenging behaviour needs to be established as their use is not without hazard. They cite litigation in the US, successfully taken, in relation to irreversible side effects of antipsychotic medication inappropriately used with people with learning disabilities.

The side effect of some antipsychoitc medication that has attracted the attention of the legal profession in America is tardive dyskinesia (involuntary movements of the tongue, lips, face, trunk and extremities). But equally worrying is the observation, again made by Ashcroft et al. (2001), in relation to another drug side effect – tardive akathesia. This creates a subjective feeling of restlessness which causes an individual to pace about and be irritable – actions which could themselves be mistaken for challenging behaviour. The manner in which side effects of medication can give rise to states which are themselves considered to be evidence of psychiatric illness has been reviewed elsewhere in relation to both tranquillisers and the new generation anti-depressants (Lynch, 2001: 61, 121).

It is of concern that the prescription of anti-psychotic medications for people with learning difficulties might be added to Lynch's list above, while other, gentler, non-medical therapies continue to be withheld for this group of people. Enabling people with learning difficulties to have full, proper, and equal access to mainstream mental health services (sometimes called generic mental health services) would be the method of choice to ensure the full range of available therapies are delivered.

Solutions for people with learning difficulties who use mental health services
How then can the situation be both safeguarded and advanced for people with learning difficulties when they confront mental health services? The answer may well be found in the development of ideas that have been around for a long time in the world of these people, their carers and their service providers that include:

- Advocacy
- Person-centred planning

Advocacy
Advocacy was a key part of *A Strategy for Equality* (Commission on the Status of People with Disabilities, 1996), the report which provided the map for developing social policy in this area. The report noted:

Advocacy is concerned with getting one's needs, wants, opinions and hopes taken seriously and acted upon. It can take a number of different forms including self-advocacy, citizen's advocacy and patient advocacy . . . the Commission believes that advocacy is essential because it allows people to participate more fully in society by expressing their own viewpoints, by participating in management and decision making and by availing of the rights to which they are entitled. (1996: 106)

To make access to such advocacy possible, the report enumerated four actions:

1   Advocacy services should be independent of service providers.
2   Self-advocacy should, where appropriate, be supplemented by the provision of citizen's advocacy. Funding for such a service should be provided by the Department of Health and Children.
3   In certain situations, the provision of independent advocacy services should be mandatory. The provision of advocacy should be incorporated into any legislation dealing with particularly vulnerable people in residential settings.
4   Funding should be provided by the Legal Aid Board to ensure that people with disabilities can employ an advocate to access expert legal representation where necessary. (Commission on the Status of People with Disabilities, 1996: 20)

Three years after the publication of this report, progress on the implementation of its recommendations was reviewed (Department of Justice, Equality and Law Reform, 1999c). This review indicated that there were almost no developments in most of the areas discussed above. In terms of independent advisory services it was noted that:

'Independent advocacy services continue to be developed and are provided by local and national user groups active on behalf of people with mental health difficulties . . . The Eastern Health Board is at present working towards provision of a patients' advocacy service' (1999: 45).

This can be interpreted as a lack of commitment by state services, leaving the work to underfunded, volunteer user groups. Not only this, but the active user groups referred to in the review were those working in mental health settings, and not the full range of self-advocates and supporting citizen advocacy for the wider sector referred to in *A Strategy for Equality*. In theory, the development and delivery of advocacy services are vested in law to Comhairle under the Comhairle Act (Department of Social and Family Affairs, 2000). In practice Comhairle, which is described as the national support agency responsible for supporting the provision of information, advice and advocacy, has commissioned a piece of research on the topic but, to date, has done little else.

A reflection document published by an organisation of people with disabilities titled: *Advocacy: A Rights Issue* (Forum for People with Disabilities, 2001) has under-scored the vulnerability of people with disabilities living in residential settings, and recommends that Ireland follow the Australian model of advocacy. This model sees advocacy not simply as a complaints and monitoring system, but as a systemic entity in society that is accountable to its users. This requires that advocacy be enabled and ensured through legislation. Advocacy did receive mention in the Disability Bill (Department of Justice, Equality and Law Reform, 2001) when it came up for debate. However, the Bill as a whole was flawed and it fell, leaving people with disabilities in Ireland without the coherently supported advocacy demanded by *A Strategy for Equality*.

Self-advocacy has been described as

> a counter-movement to state paternalism, wherein people with the label of learning difficulties conspicuously support one another to speak out against some of the most appalling examples of discrimination [it invites people] to revolt against disablement in a variety of ways, in a number of contexts, individually and collectively, with and without the support of others (Goodley, 2000: 3).

Small wonder, then, that government agencies charged with implementing policy here should be silent. In practice, there are clear differences between the 'peer advocacy' developed by mental health service users and the 'self-advocacy' that has developed around people with intellectual disabilities in Ireland. While there are groups of self-advocates with learning disabilities which hold firm to the faith of the counter-movement, the norm is for groups fostered by managements in state and voluntary body-sponsored training and living settings. Peer advocacy, meanwhile, is a dynamic champion of the rights of people subjected to psychiatric treatment (Irish Advocacy Network, 2003). In its evolution, peer advocacy has contributed a useful body of knowledge on alternatives to medical treatment for troublesome symptomatology (for instance, 'hearing voices') and this knowledge would be as usefully shared with people with learning difficulties as with anyone else.

Historically, the two approaches to advocacy have stood aloof from each other, and yet it is clear that people with a dual diagnosis have much to gain from cross-fertilisation. Part of the difficulty in achieving a meeting of minds here is reasonable suspicion on the part of peer advocates in relation to the philosophies guiding self-advocacy – where institutional self-advocacy thrives, the issues of concern may be no more radical than the menu in the canteen or the destination of the next outing. However, within the island of Ireland, peer advocacy groups north and south (working in partnership, with people from one jurisdiction on the committees of those in the other) are taking tentative steps to broaden their remit and become more inclusive – and this despite severe funding impediments (McGowan, 2003). This is encouraging, because user-led advocacy is an essential requisite of service change and development to meet the desired goal where needs are assessed and resources equitably co-ordinated and distributed.

Person-centred planning

The way in which mental health services are delivered is changing. There is a move away from the large institutions where residential patients received predominately drug-based treatments towards community-based services, which draw on a range of interventions (chemical, psychotherapeutic and group-based supports). In parallel with this shift, a user movement has been evolving which lends a new voice to an understanding of how people with mental health difficulties might be treated. This voice says that the person with a disability and/or with a mental health difficulty, defined as the same thing in Irish law (Department of Justice, Equality and Law Reform, 1999b), should be at the centre of any action plans for their future. They should also be supported to have a strong voice in any planning/treatment process developed, and should be accorded equal status with all other citizens of the state in how they are treated.

Historically, a common theme throughout service provision has been to fit the person (client, patient, user) to the service rather than the service to the person. It is an approach that has been challenged by those who have promoted concepts such as 'Person Centred Planning' and 'Personal Futures Planning'. A useful review of the current status of Person Centred Planning has been published, which provides a valuable orientation to this philosophy and its implementation (Holburn and Vietze, 2002).

The state of Alaska – like Ireland, off to the side of its continent – provides the model of best practice in relation to people with learning disabilities who use mental health services. Assets, Inc (formerly, ASETS: Alaska Specialised Education and Training Services) supports people with developmental dis-abilities or psychiatric disabilities to live, work, and learn in Anchorage (O'Brien et al., 2003). Fifty-two per cent of the service users have a 'dual diagnosis'. Simply put, this service takes on people whom other providers deem 'too difficult to serve'. O'Brien et al. (2003) understand the dilemma where those who provide services to individuals with learning disability may perceive that some people fail to make progress because they also have mental illness. Similarly, mental health service providers may decide that the same people fail to benefit from their services because they also present with a learning disability.

> From this perspective, 'too difficult' is a role created by the way a service system organises its resources. The different grids of mission, definition, knowledge, technology, accountability for funds, methods of risk management, and policy that distinguish the organisational cultures of developmental disability services

from mental health services and both systems from criminal justice services create a group of people who look anomalous from within all three perspectives. (O'Brien et al., 2003: 13)

This presents a very real trap for the service user, which Assets Inc. combat in the following ways:

- Offering a positive relationship with staff that allows people to discover and take action to pursue their hopes, dreams and personal meanings
- Providing sustained opportunities for a secure home and access to positive roles
- Offering individualised support that justifies people's trust and allows people as much autonomy and participation in community life as possible, consistent with their own safety and others' safety (O'Brien et al., 2003: 16–17)

All staff in Assets Inc. subscribe to a charter of beliefs in the people they support. These include the following beliefs that the individuals should:

- Determine their service and define what improvement means for them
- Experience discreet, non-intrusive, individualised supports of their choice
- Be respected and heard
- Be self-advocates – network with each other for support
- Get only the services they request
- Understand the obligation of service providers and expect it to be fulfilled
- Make their own decisions based on informed support

It is easy to see how all of those seven beliefs could be overridden in the current climate of Irish service provision where the primacy of decision making lies with the service provider.

Professional specialists, by definition, may focus on the problem not the person. In medical terms, they can see a hip requiring surgery followed by physiotherapy but fail to recognise a 60-year-old man who dreams of retirement and walking the hills around his home. Many medical and service professionals have become so enamoured with the assessment of quality of life and outcomes of treatments that they often miss the quality (and quantity) of the hopes and aspirations that their clients have, how much these dreams might mean and how much they need to be heard.

Reaching for these dreams and planning the route towards them are healthy human activities. These are an activities that have proved themselves through Person Centred Planning in Alaska and in many other locations. As an activity it is one that may counter ill health – as well as the deep demoralisation we call mental illness. More than this, Person Centred Planning provides the template through which persons with a learning disability who need to use psychiatric services can articulate their treatment needs. The psychiatric will was first mooted by Szasz (1987). This is a document that can be drawn up by service users supported by legal professionals. It is fashioned after the last will and living will, and is sometimes called an advanced directive. It provides a mechanism whereby individuals can lay down how they wish to be treated in the future and at those times when others consider them irrational, insane and requiring compulsory detention. Szasz argues that the 'will' accommodates the interests of both those who support and those who question or oppose compulsory detention. While such wills may be unfamiliar on the Irish scene, they have been effectively implemented in other jurisdictions (Lehmann and Kempker, 1993).

Conclusion

At the outset of this chapter it was suggested that the issues that affect people with learning difficulties have a connection to those that concern the general population in relation to mental health. This is because they are so often one and the same thing. William Anthony recently demonstrated this in a keynote address for the Year of the Person:

> We act as if the practitioner's knowledge and technology are more important than the interpersonal relationship between the practitioner and person getting help. We know this is not the case from listening to what people tell us. When asked, a majority of people who are recovering from severe mental illness will mention that a critically important contributor to their recovery is other people – people who listened to them, believed in them and supported them in numerous ways (Anthony, 2002).

Such listening can begin for people with learning disabilities, as it can for everyone, with a properly funded peer advocacy, which is supported by the structures of state to fulfil the remit it is so clearly competent to fulfil. It can be continued by the sort of planning that truly places the person at the centre of the process. Faced with legislative lethargy and service somnambulism, these are the tools for moving forward towards the achievement of a user-led comprehensive service for those with mental health problems who also have a learning disability.

Chapter 11

Crime and mental health

Vivian Geiran[1]

*'There is no more complicated or intractable a problem within criminal justice
than that posed by the needs of persons with severe mental disorders'*

(Stone, 1997: 286)

Introduction

Consideration of a topic such as mental health and crime is likely to call to
mind such high profile criminal trials as those involving John Gallagher or
Brendan O'Donnell. Both of these cases involved multiple homicides and the
subsequent trials included consideration of the issue of whether the defendants
were legally 'insane' at the time of the offences. In the Gallagher case (Hanly,
1999: 118–19), the defendant was found guilty but insane of a double homicide
in 1989. O'Donnell's trial, on the other hand, resulted in a finding of guilty of
murder (Muggivan and Muggivan, 2004). Murder trials in this category are
similar to those referred to by Guy (1869, cited in Smith, 1981: 3) as 'notorious
cases that gave rise . . . to an amount of controversy which must have carried the
fact of their acquittal or condemnation into every household in which public
affairs are heard or talked of'.

The intersection of mental health and crime undoubtedly does include
cases such as those referred to above, which have captured public imagination
and concern for generations. However, this interface also impacts in a variety
of less spectacular but no less real ways on a daily basis. Some crimes are
committed by persons already suffering from mental illness or disorder. Some
offenders[2] being managed by the justice agencies subsequently present with

---

1   The views expressed here are those of the author alone and may not necessarily reflect the views or
policies of any other bodies, including the Probation and Welfare Service and the Department of
Justice, Equality and Law Reform.

2   The term 'offender' – as in the United Nations (1990: 1) 'Tokyo Rules' on non-custodial sanctions –
is used throughout to refer to 'persons subject to prosecution, trial or the execution of a sentence' whether
they are 'suspected, accused or sentenced' and notwithstanding the fact that they might be referred to
in some circumstances as 'patients', even having been processed within the criminal justice system.

mental health problems that impact on their management. Also, crime victims and the families of victims and offenders may be affected in a variety of ways by mental health issues arising from or in conjunction with criminality. This chapter will focus in the main on the offender with mental health problems. The justice system traditionally responds to crime by detecting, prosecuting, sanctioning and managing the offender. Thus the individual offender, as well as the overall category of 'offenders' in general, are a primary focus of that system. It will not be possible to address all the elements of the mental health and crime interface in detail, particularly with regard to addictions, sexual offending and psychopathy, which are considered as falling within the remit of the mental health services.

'Insanity' and the law: a brief historical overview

The concept of 'insanity' has an important place in criminal legal history. Hanly (1999: 110) points out that:

> Broadly speaking, insanity is relevant to the criminal law in two ways. First, the defendant must be fit to plead to the charge . . . Second, where the defendant is fit to plead, the trial will proceed, but the defendant may raise the defence of insanity. The law will presume that every defendant is legally sane and, if over the age of fourteen . . . is fully accountable for his actions.

For as long as criminal law and sanctions have existed, provision has been made for those individuals deemed to be lacking in part or all of the capacity to commit crime, including those affected by mental illness. Acknowledgement of the particular position of those with mental illness as well as those with learning disabilities was included in the earliest known laws in Ireland. Based on texts from the seventh and eighth centuries, Ireland's Brehon Laws[3] employed a wide range of terms for 'persons of unsound mind' (both victims and perpetrators of crime). These terms have been described by Kelly (1988: 92), with the three most commonly used being:

- the *dásachtach* – 'the person with manic symptoms who is liable to behave in a violent and destructive manner'
- the *mer* (lit. one who is confused, deranged) – poses less threat to other people
- the *drúth* – 'appears to be a person who is mentally retarded' as well as describing the 'professional clown or buffoon whose act would include imitations of the insane'.

---

3   'Named after the travelling justices of the Celtic Christian period' (O'Mahony, 2002b).

According to Kelly (1988: 92), the Brehon Laws sought to 'protect society from the dangerously insane' and while responsibility for the actions by those described above would generally have devolved 'on his or her guardian (*conn*) who would probably be a near kinsman, such as a father or brother', a 'lenient view' would have been taken to actions committed by 'persons of unsound mind'. And in many instances the rights of those with mental illness would have taken precedence over other rights or obligations. Similarly, 'an offence committed by an insane person is normally paid for by his or her guardian, or by the person who incited the crime' (Kelly, 1988: 154), although some such actions were regarded as accidental and not actionable under the law.

In terms of modern criminal justice history, the roots of insanity as a legal defence, according to McAuley (1993: 18) can be traced back at least to the thirteenth century when Henry de Bracton 'defined the insane person as one who does not know what he is doing, who is lacking in mind and reason, and who is not far removed from the brutes' (1993: 18). Although Walker (1968: 52) cautioned against the 'misleading . . . myth that the year 1800 marked the birth of the defence of insanity', according to Hanly (1999: 110), 'it was not until *R* v. *Hadfield* (1800) that the modern defence began to take shape'. In this case, 'the defendant believed he had to die in order to save the world . . . [but] he fired a shot at the King, which was a capital offence' (Hanly, 1999: 110–11). Walker (1968: 52) acknowledged that the Hadfield case was spectacular, included expert psychiatric testimony and the outcome of that trial (a verdict of not guilty by reason of insanity) resulted in 'the first statute which expressly provided for a special verdict'. Walker (1968: 78) details several cases prior to Hadfield's in which the insanity defence was used (both successfully and unsuccessfully). He points out though, that it was not until Hadfield and the rushed legislation in response in 1800 that the 'special verdict' provided for acquittal, as well as that 'the court must order the accused "to be kept in strict custody, in such place and in such manner as the court shall seem fit, until His Majesty's pleasure be known".' However, Hanly (1999) notes that:

> The watershed, as far as modern insanity is concerned, was reached in *R* v. *M'Naghten* (1843). The defendant suffered from an insane delusion that Sir Robert Peel was persecuting him, and believed that Peel had to be killed. However, the defendant killed Peel's secretary instead. At his trial, the defendant was acquitted because of insanity. The decision caused such outrage that the House of Lords asked the Law Lords a series of questions designed to explain the defence of insanity. The answers to those questions became known as the M'Naghten Rules and they have formed the basis of the insanity defence ever since. (1999: 110)

As the Explanatory and Financial Memorandum to the Criminal Law (Insanity) Bill 2002 explains, currently 'the onus of proving insanity on the balance of probability is on the person who alleges it. If the defence is successful, the trial Judge must bring in the special verdict of "guilty but insane" as provided under the Trial of Lunatics Act, 1883, and commit the person to detention in the Central Mental Hospital.' However, McAuley (1993: 1) points out that 'the defence of insanity in Irish law has undergone considerable development' over the latter part of the twentieth century, through two stages, namely the 'theoretical acceptance of the notion of irresistible impulse by the Court of Criminal Appeal in the 1930s and the recognition of a full-blown defence of volitional insanity by the Supreme Court in 1974'.

While criminal trials of individuals charged with serious and violent crimes, including homicide, attract considerable attention, mental health issues can affect individual offenders across the full range of offending categories, which are not discrete or homogeneous. Even among the most violent types of offending, mental disorder typically presents in a small percentage of cases. For example, of the 58 murder cases disposed of in 2003, three resulted in findings of not guilty by reason of insanity. The corresponding figure for 2002 was three out of 41 cases disposed of (Courts Service, 2004: 86).

Managing offenders with mental health difficulties in the community

The issues associated with mental disorder among offenders appearing before the courts are not confined to those charged with serious offences such as homicide. The Law Reform Commission (LRC) in its consultation paper on sentencing (LRC, 1993: 41–2) acknowledged that the courts deal with cases involving accused persons presenting with a wide variety and degree of mental disorder, referring to what the Commission described to the 'inept statutory provisions . . . available to a sentencer'. It cited the Interdepartmental Committee on Mentally Ill and Maladjusted Persons (1978), which observed:

> many persons are dealt with by the courts as 'normal' offenders who are either not responsible (or not fully responsible) for the conduct charged against them or who, even if fully responsible for such conduct, are in need of psychiatric or other special treatment. The inability, or the restricted ability, of the courts to order that convicted persons receive appropriate psychiatric treatment is a grave defect in the present state of the criminal law.

The Law Reform Commission (LRC, 1993: 41) pointed out that one option 'available to a sentencer who feels that an offender should receive *psychiatric* treatment is to sentence that person to custody with a recommendation that he be sent to the Central Mental Hospital'. Within the limitations as outlined by the LRC, courts in such cases may and frequently do requisition psychiatric assessments and reports on offenders where this is indicated, warranted or suggested. Such evaluations can then be taken into account in deciding on appropriate sanctions, whether community based or custodial. While statistical data in this respect are not available, offenders placed on probation supervision would frequently have attendance at community-based psychiatric services imposed as an additional condition to a probation bond for example, where deemed appropriate. Such sentencing decisions are made in the context of judicial independence and having regard to the particular circumstances of individual cases. Data on the prevalence of mental illness or disorder among those on supervised community sanctions in this jurisdiction are not available. However, anecdotal evidence available to the author would indicate that offenders with mental health problems comprise a relatively small percentage of the average probation officer's caseload. Nevertheless, this aspect of an officer's day-to-day work may present disproportionately significant challenges.

Twenty years ago, the *Whitaker Report* (Committee of Inquiry into the Penal System, 1985) made recommendations in relation to mental health issues affecting offenders under two headings – i.e. those persons (a) appearing before the courts and (b) those in prison. The report (1985: 58) recommended that 'as a general rule, the courts should not impose a prison sentence except where no other reasonable disposal is available' and that 'the courts should explore the possibility of treatment of serious offenders with psychological/psychiatric difficulties or who are serious abusers of alcohol or drug'. The committee also (1995: 58–9) supported the recommendations of the third Henchy Report (Interdepartmental Committee on Mentally Ill and Maladjusted Persons, 1978), including that:

- Medical investigation be made available to the courts in respect of accused persons who appear to be suffering from mental disorders
- The District Court be enabled to try issues of fitness to plead and to return verdicts of 'guilty but insane' in appropriate cases, and to refer those suffering with mental disorders for out-patient care or for referral or com- mittal in appropriate residential settings
- Juries be able to make findings of diminished responsibility ('short of insanity'), thus enabling courts to decide appropriate sentences
- A special unit for detention of those offenders classified as psychopaths or sociopaths
- A Mental Care Review Body be set up to review detention of persons in designated centres and report to the appropriate court

Some commentators have called for increases in availability to the courts of community-based sanctions and diversionary programmes in respect of offenders with mental health difficulties. This would fit with the provisions of the 'Tokyo Rules' (United Nations, 1990) on non-custodial measures. Proposals have been made for the establishment of mental health courts along the lines of the United States model and similar in many respects to drug courts. Such proposals have been made by the Irish College of Psychiatrists (2003a) and by the National Forensic Mental Health Service (2003) at the CMH. Existing provision for the use of community sanctions (e.g. probation supervision with appropriate specialised case management conditions) for those with mental health issues could be strengthened without the need for entirely new court structures. Either approach would appear to be supported by the European Rules on Community Sanction and Measures (Council of Europe [CoE], 2000: Appendix 2.1). These rules (Council of Europe, 2000: Appendix 2.1) recommend, in the context of the development of varied supervised community sanctions, provision for 'treatment orders . . . for those suffering from a mental disturbance that is related to their criminal behaviour'. The European Rules also specify (Council of Europe, 1994: 7–8) that the nature of community sanctions and measures (CSMs) and the role and functions of the relevant *implementing authority* (usually a probation service managing the CSM on behalf of the court, although this is often carried out in practice in co-operation with other agencies and disciplines) should be laid down in law. Such provisions were previously proposed in the White Paper (Department of Health, 1995b: 79–81).

The National Crime Forum (1998: 154) was 'sympathetic' to the view that the assessment of mental illness among offenders should take place at the court stage of the process rather than after committal to prison. The National Economic and Social Forum (NESF, 2002: 8–12) recommended *inter alia* that:

- The use of non-custodial options in sentencing should be increased, including an expansion in the number and range of restorative justice projects (p. 9).
- 'Offenders with severe mental health problems should be diverted before or at sentencing from the prison system to appropriate alternatives' (p. 10).
- 'A strategic plan for the treatment of prisoners with mental health problems and substance abuse and/or alcohol problems should be designed and implemented in the context of Sentence Planning' (p. 10).
- 'The National Health Strategy should make specific reference to the health needs of prisoners' and 'prisoners health needs should be considered as part of their Sentence Plan' (p. 10).

Prevalence and treatment of mental disorder in the prison system

The prison became the dominant focus of penal punishment following the demise of transportation and reduced use of capital and corporal punishment in the nineteenth century, and with it came an increased prevalence of mental disorder among those in penal custody. This was especially so in the context of poor conditions and facilities, repressive regimes and a lack of association with fellow prisoners or visitors (e.g. see Carey, 2000: 94–9 with particular reference to Mountjoy Prison in Dublin). While prison still forms a major focus of sanctions for offending, much has changed for the better over more recent decades as to how those in penal custody are treated. Nevertheless, significant challenges face those with mental health issues in custody. As Peay (2002: 761) has pointed out, with reference to Britain:

> Studies of the prevalence of mental disorder in prison populations have consistently found substantial levels of disorder. Amongst the sentenced male population, Gunn et al. (1991) found that 37% had a diagnosable mental disorder. Brooke et al. (1996), looking at the remand population, found an incidence of 62%, with 5% suffering from psychosis. The 1997 national survey of psychiatric morbidity, looking at 3,000 prisoners across England and Wales (Singleton et al., 1998), found 7% of sentenced men and 10% of men on remand to have functional psychotic disorders.

Figures in relation to the corrections population (in custody or on probation or parole) in the USA indicate high prevalence of mental disorder in comparison to 'ordinary' populations. According to Ditton (1999), 16 per cent of those held in local jails, 16 per cent of state prison inmates and seven per cent of federal inmates in the USA had reported a mental illness. The figure for probationers in this study was 16 per cent. As Cowell et al. (2004: 292) indicate, 'depending on research methodology and setting, mentally ill adults represent 7% to 18% of arrested, jailed, in-prison or under-supervision populations in the United States'. However, re-offending rates for prisoners with mental health problems are apparently generally 'no higher than those for any other group of offender' (Harper and Chitty, 2004: 23).

Comparable data on similar categories of person in this jurisdiction are not as readily available in such detail. However, a number of relevant studies have been carried out in recent years. Echoing the earlier comment by Stone (1997: 286), research by the Centre for Health Promotion Studies (CHPS, 2000: 59) on various aspects of healthcare in prisons observed that 'mental health is one of the outstanding health care issues within the Irish prison population . . . Thirty seven per cent of male prisoners . . . and 64% of female prisoners described themselves as moderately or extremely anxious/depressed' and that 'nearly half of the men and 75% of the women . . . may be significantly in need of psychiatric treatment'. Smith et al. (1996, cited in NESF, 2002: 42) 'found higher rates of mental illness [in a sample of prisoners committed to Mountjoy Prison] than would be expected in the general population', finding that '4% of those assessed had a major mental illness (such as schizophrenia) and a further 7% had some psychiatric disorder, such as a panic disorder. A further 46% of cases were found to be dependent on illicit drugs and/or alcohol.' O'Mahony's study of a sample of prisoners in Mountjoy prison for males in Dublin (1997: 115) had earlier reported high rates of attendance with psychiatrists, transfer to the Central Mental Hospital (CMH), use of medication and self-harm.

Management of prisoners[4] with mental health difficulties

The 1947 Prison Rules (Department of Justice, 1947) deal with all aspects of the management and operation of prisons in this jurisdiction up to the present. They include, *inter alia*, provisions regarding medical examination on reception into penal custody (11.9) and on transfer between institutions (11.16), the use of padded cells, the role of prison chaplains in monitoring prisoners' mental status (IV.165), and the role of the 'medical officer' (physician) in relation to the mental health of prisoners. The latter specifically includes monitoring and reporting to the Governor and/or Minister instances where 'the mental state of any prisoner is becoming impaired or enfeebled', and keeping 'statistics of sickness, mortality, removal on medical grounds, insanity, suicide, and hospital treatment' (v.172–88). The Prison Rules refer to and set out the duties of a number of named officials including the governor, custodial personnel, chaplain and medical officer (physician), but not to a number of other professionals that have since acquired roles in prison regimes, including probation officers and psychologists, among others. At the time of writing, revised prison rules are being prepared. It is expected that they will also be augmented by updated European Prison Rules, an earlier version having been published in 1987 (Council of Europe, 1987).

Under the heading 'Special Categories of Offenders', the Whitaker Report (Committee of Inquiry into the Penal System, 1985: 85–8) considered psychiatric services for offenders in penal custody and made a number of recommendations. As well as proposing specific measures for improved treatment for alcohol and drug abuse, and for those prisoners with learning disabilities and sex offenders, the committee recognised that the accommodation and treatment of 'high security risk prisoners suffering from psychiatric problems poses particular problems'. It recommended that a 'small psychiatric unit should be established in Portlaoise Prison' for such prisoners. It is likely that this recommendation

---

4   Used to refer to those 'offenders' detained in custody, whether in prison or the CMH.

was linked to the presence of a relatively high number of paramilitary prisoners at the time of the Whitaker investigation. The report (1985: 88) also expressed the view that 'there are too many long stay patients in the Central Mental Hospital . . . who could be treated effectively in Health Board psychiatric hospitals' and recommended 'that these patients be transferred accordingly to free the resources of the Central Mental Hospital' for those the committee believed should be catered for at Dundrum. These included:

- the normal run of prisoners requiring treatment for psychiatric disorders
- sociopaths/psychopaths
- sex offenders
- drug/alcohol abusers who require specialist treatment (appropriately in the new drug unit)

The Irish Prison Service (IPS) has a strategic objective to 'ensure medical and psychiatric care for prisoners to a standard consistent with that which applies in the community generally' (IPS, 2003: 95). The Service had previously reported difficulties recruiting and retaining 'a variety of health care professionals to provide services within the prison system' (IPS, 2001: 15). By 2002, however, a Director of Regimes had been appointed, supporting a 'multi-faceted approach to re-balancing the Service's custodial and care/rehabilitation functions' (IPS, 2003: 27). Psychiatric services are supplied to prisons outside Dublin by visiting psychiatrists generally employed by local health boards. 'Offenders who, in the opinion of the psychiatrist and the Prison Doctor, are in need of in-patient treatment, may be transferred by Ministerial Order to either the Central Mental Hospital or a District Mental Hospital. In practice, such transfers occur to the Central Mental Hospital' (IPS, 2001: 16).

The Central Mental Hospital is the only secure forensic hospital in Ireland and provides a forensic psychiatric service for the entire country, with 'in-patient care . . . provided at the eighty-eight-bed . . . Hospital' at Dundrum (Inspector of Mental Hospitals, 2003: 45).

It was established under the provisions of the Central Criminal Lunatic Asylum (Ireland) Act, 1845. The hospital provides psychiatric care in conditions of medium and high security for patients transferred from the prison system, those found unfit to plead or guilty but insane, and those transferred from local area mental health services under Section 207 or 208 of the Mental Treatment Act, 1945. Approximately 1.3% of all committals to prisons are transferred to the CMH, as compared to 0.2% in the UK and 0.8% in Holland. The CMH provides forensic psychiatric assessment, treatment and rehabilitation for all the health boards in the country and, in addition, provides the Irish prison population with an assessment and treatment service in the greater Dublin region. The hospital was managed by the Department of Health up to 1972 and from 1972 by the Eastern Health Board. With the rearrangement of the health services in the eastern region, responsibility for its management has transferred to the East Coast Area Health Board. (Inspector of Mental Hospitals, 2003: 47)

A total of 117 prisoners (109 men and eight women) were transferred from prisons to the CMH in 1983 (Department of Justice, 1983: 23). In 1990, the figure was 345 (including 49 women) (Department of Justice, 1990; 46). Comparable statistics are not presented in more recent annual reports of the Irish Prison Service. There was apparently a total of 136 admissions of all categories, including those transferred from prisons, to the CMH in 2001 (Inspector of Mental Hospitals, 2003: 46).

A Director of Prison Medical Services was appointed in 1990. This had been recommended in the *Whitaker Report*. Subsequently, the Department of Justice (1994) published an action plan for the development of services dealing with the management of offenders, primarily in relation to the penal system. The objectives of the prison medical services as set out in that document included: primary health care provision, standards of treatment and staffing, links with services in the community and involvement of prisoners in service planning and delivery. The plan highlighted continuing difficulties in the provision of services to prisoners (including the inadequacy of the 1947 Prison Rules, the need to improve arrangements in relation to general medical and psychiatric services in prisons, the absence of qualified nurses in the prison service, and inadequate number of beds available for prisoners in the CMH) and set priority targets for action. Themes developed in the 1994 plan, including that custodial sentences should be the sanction of last resort, were repeated in the subsequent discussion paper (Department of Justice, 1997) and Departmental strategy statements (e.g. Department of Justice, Equality and Law Reform, 2003).

An Inspector of Prisons and Places of Detention, Mr Justice Dermot Kinlen, was appointed in April 2002. Inspections include consideration of the 'health, safety and well-being of prisoners' (Inspector of Prisons and Places of Detention, 2004: 13). In his reports, the Inspector has considered mental health issues affecting prisoners, including the practice of conveying prisoners to the CMH for psychiatric treatment instead of using facilities nearer to individual prisons, the operation of multi-disciplinary suicide prevention groups in prisons, forensic psychiatrist staffing levels in prisons, mental health legislation and the general organisation of psychiatric services for prisoners.

Recent policy and legislation

The report of the Study Group on the Development of the Psychiatric Services, *The Psychiatric Services: Planning for the Future* (Study Group, 1984) was published two decades ago. Its purpose was to provide the blueprint for the future development of psychiatric services in Ireland. Significant recommendations of the report related to the need to develop a comprehensive, sectorised, community-oriented psychiatric service in Ireland. The report envisaged psychiatric services throughout the state that would include adequate provision for prevention and early identification of illness, assessment, diagnostic and treatment services, in-patient and day care, out-patient treatment, community residences, and rehabilitation and training, all to be provided by multi-disciplinary teams in geographically bounded sectors of population. *Planning for the Future* (Study Group, 1984) did not specifically address issues related to mental health and crime *per se*. A Green Paper on Mental Health (Department of Health, 1992) did include discussion of a range of issues affecting forensic psychiatric services in this jurisdiction, and set out Government thinking on issues such as the need for new legislation (specifically in relation to 'criminal insanity'), providing the courts with a wider range of options to deal with mentally ill offenders and clarifying the role of the CMH, as well as raising a number of questions for discussion with a view to implementing appropriate change in these areas.

The White Paper that followed (Department of Health, 1995b: 66–81) similarly referred to 'Mentally Disordered Persons before the Courts and in Custody'. Proposals (1995: 79–81) included changes in mental health legislation on criminal insanity. It further recommended that persons with a mental disorder appearing before the courts should be treated with minimal formality, with structured assessment and diversion to community-based programmes where appropriate, or alternatively residential treatment in prison or a special psychiatric facility as appropriate. The White Paper also recommended that the CMH and other specially designated psychiatric centres be utilised for prisoners who commit serious offences and are dangerous, and that those convicted of minor offences and not posing issues of public safety, be referred to other centres for treatment where appropriate,

Given the widespread acceptance that the criminal legislation on insanity and related matters was in need of modernisation, the publication of the Criminal Justice (Mental Disorder) Bill 1996 heralded change in this area. While that Bill has since been superseded, mental health legislation in Ireland was updated significantly by the Mental Health Act 2001. This statute (Section 3) defines 'mental disorder' as including 'mental illness, severe dementia or significant intellectual disability' and details the elements of these definitions. The legislation in relation to the mental health of those who may have committed offences and are appearing before the courts is to be further updated by the Criminal Law (Insanity) Bill 2002 (before the Oireachtas at the time of writing). The Bill's explanatory memorandum acknowledges the 'development of modern psychiatry and greater understanding of the underlying causes of mental illness' and recognises that 'this area of the criminal law needs clarification and development'. It describes a function of the new legislation as being to draw up 'appropriate rules to govern the criminal responsibility of mentally ill persons who may have committed offences' and the purpose of the Bill as being 'to clarify, modernise and reform the law on criminal insanity and fitness to be tried and on related issues; and, to bring it into line with the jurisprudence of the European Convention on Human Rights'. The European Convention on Human Rights was passed into law in 2003.

This Bill includes a definition of 'mental disorder', enables the Minister for Health and Children to designate psychiatric centres (including prisons or parts of prisons) for the reception, detention, care and treatment of persons committed under this legislation, clarification of 'unfitness to be tried' (to replace the current concept of fitness to plead) and verdicts of 'not guilty by reason of insanity' and 'diminished responsibility' (in murder cases). It also provides for disposal of cases before the courts in which such findings are made, as well as the establishment of an independent Mental Health Review Board to regularly 'review . . . the detention of persons found not guilty by reason of insanity or unfit to be tried, who have been detained in a designated centre by order of a court'. Although the 2002 Bill has been widely welcomed, there have been some concerns expressed and suggestions made for amendments (e.g. Bergin and Hunter, 2003). At the time of writing, this piece of legislation has yet to pass all stages before the Oireachtas.

Key issues for further consideration

Significant issues which affect services for offenders with mental disorders and impact on policy developments are discussed in this section.

Public perceptions and information on mental illness and offending

The perception that a significant percentage of persons with mental health problems are dangerous and given to extreme violence has been mentioned already. Such perception may be fuelled (Wahl, 2003) by media representations, for example a newspaper report that 'a man with a history of mental illness was arrested in connection with . . . attacks' in which 'a knife-wielding man killed one person and critically injured five others . . . in a series of apparently random stabbings across North London' (*The Irish Times*, 24 December 2004). Such reports, while factual, may contribute to a 'pejorative perception that people who commit an act of homicide are "mad" or suffering from some form of mental illness, or at least mentally disordered in some way' (Dooley, 1995: 26). This perception is not borne out statistically by the available research evidence. Dooley (1995, 28) points out that of over twenty years of homicide cases studied in Ireland, only 5.1 per cent (N = 31) of the total involved 'psychiatric verdicts brought in by the courts' while 'in a small number of cases a defendant was considered unfit to plead'. It should be noted, however, that Dooley points to 'the lack of any form of diminished responsibility (on the basis of psychiatric disorder) verdict in Irish law' as contributing to the relatively low level of psychiatric verdicts as compared to other jurisdictions such as Britain where, according to Dooley (1995: 28), around 15 per cent of homicide convictions are in this category. Where they persist, such attitudes militate against service provision to offenders and especially against their social inclusion and integration in the community.

Dual diagnosis, criminalisation and trans-institutionalisation of the mentally ill

Dual diagnosis refers to the co-existence of mental disorder and drug or alcohol dependence. Such co-existence can lead to a perceived 'vicious circle' of disputed prioritisation of the two elements of the dual diagnosis and a reluctance to treat one set of issues until the other is adequately addressed. Dual diagnosis presents particular difficulty for primarily single focus and specialised services, which may not cater for simultaneous treatment of other problems. Difficulties can be further exacerbated when, as is often the situation, an individual at the centre of a dual diagnosis is also identified as an offender, as well as perhaps facing other complicating problems such as homelessness, physical ill-health or disability. Until recently, this phenomenon had received little research attention in this jurisdiction. Now MacGabhann et al. (2004) have carried out research on the issues associated with dual diagnosis. This should contribute to the recognition of the issues involved and may lead to more effective responses.

The concept of the 'revolving door' of transinstitutionalisation has been applied to situations where individual service users are 'recycled' into and out of institutional services, whether psychiatric – including addictions – or penal. The phenomenon in question, also referred to as 'transcarceration', refers to the 'ongoing routing of mentally ill offenders to and from the mental health and the criminal justice systems' (Arrigo, 2001: 162). There is a view that in some situations psychiatric treatment may be accessed more readily if the individual is referred through the justice system. Hartwell (2004: 95) states that:

> The differences between offenders with mental illness and those with mental illness and substance abuse problems, the dually diagnosed, are pronounced. The dually diagnosed are more likely to be serving sentences related to their substance

use (public order offences, property crimes and drug-dealing offences). They are also more likely to be homeless on release, violate probation . . . and recidivate to correctional custody.

The multiple problems presented by this group need to be addressed in combination. Redmond in chapter 12 on homelessness addresses some of these issues in more detail.

Focus on what works – care or control? punishment or treatment?

There has been a considerable amount of research carried out over the past decade or so into what works in reducing re-offending among offenders (Harper and Chitty, 2004). This enquiry 'has been successful in identifying risk factors which are associated with re-offending, including education, employment, accommodation, substance misuse, mental health and social networks problems (as well as thinking and behaviour)' (Harper and Chitty, 2004: 29). Harper and Chitty (2004: 64) also note that 'mental health problems are likely to impede the ability of both prisoners and probationers to access and properly engage in offending related programmes.' There is clearly a need for further research into what works best in reducing re-offending with mentally disordered offenders, the relative impact of supervision in the community and comparisons with custodial options, and the appropriateness of standardised offending behaviour (and other) programmes – both in the community and in custody – with such offenders.

The Committee of Inquiry into the Penal System (1985: 85) suggested that 'the emphasis in prison psychiatry should be to promote the mental health of the prisoners rather than the broader aim of attempting to reform them'. According to the Law Reform Commission (LRC, 1996: 19): 'Rehabilitation clearly conflicts on occasion with the principle of just deserts' and imprisonment imposed on 'an offender who is mentally disturbed where the offending behaviour has been very serious . . . may be counter-productive . . . in terms of rehabilitation and may even in some cases reinforce criminal tendencies.' The Centre for Health Promotion Studies (CHPS, 2000: 59) emphasised that 'the burden of mental ill-health in Irish prisons' and 'the disabling effects of mental illness and the high levels of distress must be reduced in order to maximise the rehabilitative potential of a prison sentence'. The NESF (2002: 42) also acknowledged 'concerns about the suitability of normal prison accommodation for prisoners with mental health difficulties' and referred to similar concerns expressed by other bodies in this regard (Advisory Group on Prison Deaths, 1991: 78; Council of Europe CPT, 1999: 35). This issue will require more attention to optimise both community-based and custodial sanctions and treatment.

Personality disorder and psychopathy
The problems associated with those classified as having a personality disorder
and psychopathy have been acknowledged as far back as the Commission of
Inquiry on Mental Illness, 1966: 96–8) and taken up in Henchy Report
(Interdepartmental Committee, 1978) and Whitaker Report (Committee of
Enquiry into the Penal System, 1985). There is evidence that of those offenders
who present with some form of mental disorder, those with psychopathic or
personality disorders are relatively more dangerous and more likely to offend
than those in other categories. For example, Jamieson and Taylor (2004: 783)
found that of a sample of persons released from high security hospitals, 'people
with personality disorder were seven times more likely than people with mental
illness to be convicted of a serious offence after discharge'. As Jamieson and
Taylor (2004: 783) comment, 'when people with a major mental disorder
[including mental illness, psychopathic disorder *inter alia*] are thought to pose
a high risk to others, particularly after conviction for a serious offence, they are
generally detained in one of the three high security (special) hospitals in
England'. The same authors (2004: 784) also point out that 'the personality
disorders are more or less coterminous with the legal category of psychopathic
disorder'. I am aware of anecdotal evidence of reluctance in services in this
jurisdiction to deal with offenders diagnosed as personality disordered or
psychopathic as opposed to mentally ill, which can result in a perception by
some professionals that they are being left to 'pick up the pieces' in such
instances. This observation is echoed by the Inspector of Prisons and Places of
Detention (2004: 73), who, while praising the dedication of those providing
services at the CMH, observes that they 'will not take in people who merely
have personality disorders.'

Conclusion

'Arguably, the weakest of those brought before the courts in criminal matters
are the mentally ill' (Byrne et al., 1981: 131). This chapter has outlined the
complex nature of the issues involved in a debate that can be dominated by a
small number of high profile, serious, yet statistically unrepresentative cases.
Far more common are the offenders with mental health problems before the
courts, on probation supervision or in custody arising from relatively less
serious charges. Although only a small percentage of serious violent crime is
committed by persons with mental illness, there is some evidence that those
offenders presenting with personality disorder or psychopathy pose disproportionate challenges. While there is a long history of justice system responses to
these issues, at present much of the relevant legislation dates back to the nineteenth century, with the 1945 Mental Treatment Act still occupying a central

place in service provision. Research evidence has shown that there is a high prevalence of mental illness among those in prison and on community sanctions. Challenges arising are further complicated in cases involving dual diagnoses and co-existence of other serious issues such as homelessness. The Department of Justice, Equality and Law Reform (2003: 47) has acknowledged the 'need to take innovative and comprehensive approaches to meet the challenges presented by certain types of offenders' including those 'who are mentally ill'. The Department's Strategy Statement (2003: 47) goes on to state that the 'Criminal Justice (Insanity) Bill will reform the process by which the criminal law will deal with mentally ill offenders'. A series of studies and reports of inquiry have acknowledged the difficulties inherent in responses to date and have pointed to clear areas for improvement (e.g. National Crime Forum, 1998: 154; Mental Health Commission, 2004a). It seems clear that despite new legislation and a case being made for improved resourcing, as with so many other 'cross-cutting' issues, enhanced interagency and multi-disciplinary co-ordination of services will be required to maximise the effectiveness of any legislative, structural and service developments. Diversion into appropriate treatment prior to any involvement with or by the justice agencies would appear to hold out most promise. Where criminal justice system involvement becomes inevitable, non-custodial responses are most appropriate, where applicable, with the use of custody being the sanction of last resort – not the 'default' option for whatever reason.

Recommended reading

Department of Health (1995b) *White Paper: A New Mental Health Act.* Dublin: Stationery Office.

Peay, J. (2002) 'Mentally disordered offenders, mental health, and crime', in Maguire, M., Morgan, R. and Reiner, R. (eds), *The Oxford Handbook of Criminology*, 3rd edn. Oxford: Oxford University Press.

McAuley, F. (1993) *Insanity, Psychiatry and Criminal Responsibility.* Dublin: Round Hall.

NESF (2002) *Reintegration of Prisoners*, Forum Report no. 22. Dublin: NESF.

Chapter 12

Homelessness and mental health

Bairbre Redmond

*'People who are mentally ill and homeless are among the most
destitute and neglected people in our society'*
(McKeown, 1999: 4)

People who are homeless are faced with a way of life that is both physically
exhausting and psychologically distressing and, from the nature of the life they
have to lead, are particularly vulnerable to physical and mental health problems
(O'Sullivan, 1996: 8). However, homelessness and mental illness are bound
together in a more complex equation and many people with pre-existing
mental health problems may also find themselves more vulnerable to becoming
homeless. McKeown (1999: 7) notes that while no more than ten per cent of the
Irish population suffer from mental health problems, between a quarter and a
half of the Irish homeless population have mental illness or are addicted to
alcohol or drugs. Individuals leaving institutional settings such as prison, child
care and long-term hospital care (particularly psychiatric care) are also known
to be at greater risk of homelessness (Daly, 1993; Kellegher et al., 2000). Such
individuals may have few family members to support them on their discharge
and, indeed, some of their reasons for needing care or detention systems in the
first place may have been based on poor family support and/or significant
psychological difficulties.

This chapter looks at some of the issues and the policy responses relating to
homelessness for those with mental health difficulties. It looks at the impact of
the closure of large psychiatric institutions and the subsequent deinstutionalisation on those with mental health problems into what was termed 'care in
the community'. The chapter examines the development of policies targeting
both homelessness and mental health, and also focuses on specific groups who
are vulnerable to homelessness and mental illness including those with drug
and alcohol problems and children and young adults either living in homeless
families or leaving state care. Research indicates that many individuals who are
homeless with mental health problems end up in trouble with the law and

many recently released prisoners enter the homeless population. While this particular cohort is not explored in this chapter, a discussion of the issues facing offenders with mental illness can be found in chapter 11.

Historical overview of mental health and homelessness

In order to understand the growing numbers of people with mental health problems, both nationally and internationally, who become homeless it is necessary to examine the impact of deinstitutionalisation. Robins notes that in Ireland many psychiatric institutions were founded from the late eighteenth century onwards because of the growing need 'to confine the many disturbed and uncontrolled persons who were wandering abroad' (Robins, 1986: 37). Timms (1993) notes that psychiatric studies from the early twentieth century recognised that many admissions to psychiatric institutions were of men who had no fixed abode, many of whom were suffering from schizophrenia. Little was done to explore this connection and, in the main, most people with mental health difficulties were cared for, in the long term, in institutional settings.

From the late 1950s onwards there was growing political pressure to move services – for those with mental health problems and for those with disability – out of institutions and into smaller, community settings. Such moves were not only in response to the demands for better quality care, but were also related to the escalating costs of running large institutions and the belief that services could be provided at less cost within the community (Mansell and Ericsson, 1996; Walker, 1993). New approaches for those with mental illness, such as psychotherapy and new drug treatments, particularly the use of the chlorpromazine group of drugs, had a major impact on the treatment of schizophrenia and other psychotic disorders. While these new therapies did not bring about a lasting cure, 'it was now possible to consider alternatives to the deeply rooted policies of isolation and confinement' (Robins, 1986: 198). For many with mental health difficulties, the move into care within the community offered the potential for new freedoms and the chance of leading far more normal lives.

In the United Kingdom, the Report of the 1954–7 Royal Commission on the Law relating to Mental Illness and Mental Deficiency, the Percy Report (Departments of State and Official Bodies and Royal Commission on the Law Relating to Mental Illness and Mental Deficiency, 1957) marked a turning point in the care of those with mental illness, moving from asylum-based care to care in community settings (Timms, 1993; Crane, 1999). Timms (1993) notes that the decline in psychiatric beds in the United Kingdom's National Health Service (NHS) started in 1954. In the past ten years, the average daily number of NHS beds available for mental illness in England has almost halved (UK, Department of Health, 2003). In the United States, the enactment of the

Mental Retardation Facilities and Community Mental Health Centres Construction Act (1963) heralded similar changes, and, during the period 1963 to 1980, the numbers in public psychiatric hospitals in the US declined from 504,000 to 138,000 (Merwin and Ochberg, 1983: 96).

The Irish government's policies for setting up a modern, community-based mental health service were first revealed in the *Commission of Inquiry into Mental Illness* (Department of Health, 1966) and further developed in the *The Psychiatric Services: Planning for the Future* (Department of Health, 1984). Both documents proposed the establishment of psychiatric units in general hospitals as well as locally based hostels, community residences and smaller day hospitals and centres where individuals could receive support and treatment near to home. These proposed changes began to be introduced, with the most obvious result being the closures of the large psychiatric hospitals. The numbers of patients in these hospitals began to decline from a peak of 21,075 in 1958. In 1983 the total mental hospital population in Ireland had fallen to 12,802 and by 2001 it was approximately 4,000 (Department of Health, 1984; Robins, 1986; Daly and Walsh, 2002). What was less in evidence was the establishment of a well co-ordinated, flexible community-based response for those with mental health difficulties (Fernandez, 1996). The Green Paper on Mental Health (Department of Health, 1992) acknowledged the need for greater co-ordination and integration of services. In their submission to the Expert Group on Mental Health Policy, the Irish College of Psychiatrists (2004b) noted that the targets set out in *The Psychiatric Services: Planning for the Future* (Department of Health, 1984) had not been met over the previous twenty years. This report highlighted uneven service provision between health board areas in term of community-based mental health service provision and noted that many psychiatric day hospitals were generally failing to provide a service for acutely ill patients. Harvey comments that in all the reforms of the mental health service in the last thirty years, the needs of those who are homeless or in danger of becoming homeless have been largely ignored (1998: 14–15).

The connection between the closure of larger psychiatric hospitals and the increasing number of people with mental illness who are homeless can often been seen as a simple one. Yet for those who have been discharged, it is often not the absence of the larger institution to return to that precipitates them into homelessness. Rather, what are lacking are good, community-based alternative services which are flexible enough to meet the needs of individuals whose mental health put them at risk of homelessness. Crane (1999: 71) also points out that in Britain and the United States many individuals with mental illness who are currently homeless have never been hospitalised. There is also evidence (Appleby, 1985; Snow and Anderson, 1993; Rosenthal, 1994) that many of the homeless mentally ill who had been hospitalised were not long-stay patients, rather their contact with the services was in the form of frequent brief

admissions. When the long-stay hospitals closed, a source of temporary accommodation at times of crisis for many individuals with fragile mental health
patterns was taken away – such crisis accommodation was not adequately
replaced within community settings

> The rise in homelessness in the 1980s has often been linked to deinstiutional-
> isation of psychiatric patients into the community. In Ireland, the evidence is less
> that discharged former long-stay patients became homeless but rather that the
> reduction of long-stay beds closed off what in effect was a residual social accom-
> modation performed by long-stay psychiatric hospitals. (Harvey, 1998: 4)

Social policy and the homeless mentally ill

Irish policy responses to those who are mentally ill and homeless have been
patchy and Harvey has noted that the level of legislative protection for
homeless people in Ireland can be seen as low by European standards (1998: 11).
Moreover, the responsibility for those with mental illness who are homeless
spans a number of governmental departments including housing, health,
justice and child and family welfare. This results in a situation in which no one
department is responsible for the needs of this particular group and, in the main,
their needs have been relegated to a sub-set of policies and services designed
either to address homelessness, or to those designed to tackle mental health
issues or, in some cases, child care and protection services. Because of such
cross-departmental involvement, a large number of policy documents and
pieces of state legislation have been produced that deal with homelessness and
mental health. Most of these documents refer tangentially to those with mental
illness who become homeless and table 12.1 provides a brief summary of the
policy and legislation that touches, albeit briefly, on the needs of those with
mental illness who become homeless.

McKeown proposes that, in terms of policy and service delivery, the
homeless mentally ill should be primarily regarded as disabled 'since it is their
mental illness . . . which is the primary influence on their lives' (1999: 3).
However, policies directed at mental health have not addressed the problems of
the mentally ill homeless, despite repeated mention of the needs of this cohort
in the Annual Reports of the Inspector of Mental Hospitals. In his final report
the Inspector stated that 'it was clear that there needed to be a concerted,
global, integrated and coordinated response of multidisciplinary nature to the
problem [of homelessness and mental illness] which was currently lacking'
(Walsh, 2004: 11). Fernandez (1996: 225) notes that in *The Psychiatric Services:
Planning for the Future* (Department of Health, 1984), an important policy
document that addressed the needs of the mentally ill in Ireland, a mere 26 lines

Table 12.1 **Policy and legislation relating to homelessness and mental health**

Commission of Enquiry into Mental Illness (Department of Health, 1966)	Blueprint of modern mental health service outlined including proposals to care for those with mental illness in the community. Populations in large psychiatric hospitals begin to decline
The Psychiatric Services: Planning for the Future (Department of Health, 1984)	Establishment of psychiatric units in general hospitals as well as locally based hostels, community residences and smaller day hospitals and centres. Further decline in numbers in large psychiatric hospitals
Housing Act 1988 Homeless Persons Act	Section 2 of the Act provided the first legal definition of homelessness in Ireland. For the first time Section 10 of the Act placed responsibility on housing authorities to provide accommodation to homeless people.
Child Care Act 1991	Section 5 of the Act put a statutory obligation on health boards to provide accommodation to homeless children
Green Paper on Mental Health (Department of Health, 1992)	Aimed to provide a comprehensive and community oriented psychiatric service
Counted In (Williams and O'Connor, 1999)	First comprehensive census of homeless population in Dublin. Similar census subsequently carried out in 2002
National Children's Strategy (Department of Health and Children, 2000a)	Identified the development of a national strategy on youth homelessness as a priority in addressing homelessness among young people
Homelessness: An Integrated Strategy (Department of the Environment and Local Government, 2000)	Cross-departmental report relating to accommodation, heath, welfare and educational issues and preventive strategies
Youth Homelessness Strategy (Department of Health and Children, 2001g)	Government strategy aimed at achieving a more co-ordinated and planned approach to tackling the issue of youth homelessness.
Mental Health Act 2001	Brought Irish laws into line with the international obligations for the protection of the rights of people who require compulsory psychiatric admission and treatment

National Health Strategy – *Quality and Fairness* (Department of Health and Children, 2001b)	To ensure equity, people-centredness, quality and accountability in health policy and services.
Homelessness Preventative Strategy (Department of the Environment and Local Government, 2002)	Cross-departmental government strategy to prevent homelessness among those leaving hospitals, mental hospitals, childcare and prison.
Mental Health Commission 2002	Independent group established by Mental Health Act 2001 to encourage and maintain high standards and good practice in the area of mental health.
Expert group on Mental Health Policy, 2003	Expert Group established to examine all aspects of mental health care and treatment for next ten years. Group will report in 2005.

of its 138 pages focused on the needs of the homeless. Likewise, Amnesty International has expressed concern that planning appropriate effective responses for the homeless with mental illness may be seriously hampered by the lack of government data on service provision and needs analyses (Crowley, 2003: 47).

In the Amnesty International report, *Mental Illness: The Neglected Quarter*, Crowley also notes that in Ireland voluntary organisations are filling gaps in government policy implementation, not only in relation to service provision, but also in research and data collection (2003: 10). Certainly organisations such as Focus Ireland (Focus Ireland et al., 2000; Kellegher et al., 2000), the Simon Community (Collins and McKeown, 1992; Dublin Simon Community, 2003a) and Merchant's Quay Project (Cox and Lawless, 1999) have produced critically important data and policy analysis on services for the homeless with mental illness. Part of the rationale for the establishment of the Homeless Agency in 2000 was to create a partnership structure for homeless services, bringing together the voluntary and statutory agencies responsible for planning, funding and delivering services to people who are homeless. Established as part of the government strategy on homelessness, the Homeless Agency is responsible for the management and co-ordination of services to people who are homeless in the Dublin area and for the implementation of agreed action plans which aim to eliminate homelessness in the capital by 2010. The Homeless Agency's remit was also formed by two important policy documents, *Homelessness: An Integrated Strategy* (Department of the Environment and Local Government, 2000) and the *Homelessness Preventative Strategy* (Department of the Environment and Local Government, 2002), both of which attempted to rationalise and co-ordinate the statutory and voluntary homeless services and to create a partnership-based approach to further planning in the area.

Profile of the homeless with mental illness

Amnesty International's report on homelessness and mental health in Ireland notes that the numbers of people homeless in Ireland is a matter of some debate (Crowley 2003: 15). Certainly up to the late 1990s little reliable data have been available on the number who are homeless, let alone the numbers of those amongst them who have mental health difficulties. O'Sullivan (1996: 3–5) maintains that the Irish state has consistently attempted to minimise the numbers of those who were homeless in Ireland and that knowledge about the characteristics of the homeless population in this country was largely non-existent. Harvey (1998: 4) contends that the levels of mental illness in the homeless population can range from three per cent to 91 per cent, depending on the methodologies and definition used and the groups studied. Fernandez, who puts the number of homeless with mental illness at 75 per cent, cautions that 'estimates vary depending on one's definition of homelessness and on other less scientific influences shaded by consideration of a political or campaigning nature' (cited in Crowley, 2003: 18).

The characteristics of those who are homeless with mental health problems are also difficult to measure, although it is clear that the profile of the general homeless population is changing. Cleary and Prizeman (1998: 11) note that, from both Irish and international data, homeless people are predominantly male, single (or separated) and middle-aged. They also note that these trends are changing with a move towards higher numbers of women, children and young adults in the homeless population. *Counted in 2002* (Williams and Gorby, 2002), the most recent census of the homeless population in Dublin noted that homeless men have a much higher tendency to sleep rough than women, while homeless women (particularly women with children) are more likely to make use of bed & breakfast accommodation (Williams and Gorby, 2002: 30–1). We shall look at issues for the homeless mentally ill population in general and will focus on issues for groups becoming more prevalent in this population such as women, children and young single adults.

Table 12.2 summarises a number of Irish studies that have attempted to measure the mental health of different cohorts of those who are homeless. The table also shows the reasons for the different groups' entry into homelessness, the so-called 'pathways to homelessness'.

Table 12.2 **Incidences of mental illness and pathways to homelessness**

Author/s	Population studies	Evidence of mental health problems	Reasons for becoming homeless
Holohan (1997)	502 people living in hostels, b & bs and sleeping rough	39% had chronic psychiatric problems	Drug/alcohol abuse Relationship problems Financial problems Eviction
Cleary and Prizeman (1998)	50 people attending a drop-in centre for out of-home people (80% male)	40% had psychiatric illness	Family problems Lack of accommodation Substance abuse Psychiatric illness
Cox & Lawless (1999)	53 out-of-home drug users presenting at a contact centre	78% suffered from depression 46% reported anxiety 58% felt unable to cope	Drug use Family conflict Relationship breakdown Money problems
Feeney et al. (2000)	171 hostel-dwelling men	64% with mental health problems	Separation from wife/partner Addiction problems Problems with previous accommodation Family problems
Houghton and Hickey (2000)	1202 households placed in emergency b & b accommodation in 1999	20% gave mental or physical health problems as their main or secondary reasons for homelessness	Family conflict Eviction Drug addiction
Smith et al. (2001)	100 homeless women (including 82 mothers) living in b&b and hostel accommodation	73% of women reported mental health problems	Lack of affordable accommodation Domestic violence Family problems Addiction problems
Eastern Regional Health Authority (2002a)	158 children presenting to Regional health boards as homeless in 2000	Mental health not measured	Family problems Emotional/behavioural difficulties Physical abuse Child abandoned
Focus Ireland et al. (2000)	14 Families (previously homeless) in transitional housing with Focus Ireland	29% of the mothers had mental health problems. 38% of children tested had mental health difficulties.	Relationship difficulties Drug dependency Domestic violence

Source: Adapted from Focus Ireland (2003: 24)

Connections between homelessness and mental illness

Pre-existing mental illness

One of the most fundamental debates on homelessness and mental health is whether mental illness predates and causes homelessness or whether the stress of being homeless causes mental health problems. Fernandez (2003), often a lone voice calling for services for the homeless mentally ill in Ireland, highlights the need to differentiate between mental health problems brought about by homeless and mental illness which may be a factor in becoming and remaining homeless. The foregoing discussion on the impact of deinstutionalisation implies that a pre-existing mental illness increases the chance of becoming homeless, particularly when appropraite mental health services have not been put in place. Crane (1999) studied over 200 homeless men and women in four cities in the UK and found that over 41 per cent had experienced mental health problems before they became homeless. Of this group, some became homeless owing to the breakdown of families or social supports, primarily the death of one or both parents who had been their carers. Others became homeless following a significantly stressful life event, marital breakup, or when their existing mental illness became more severe and debilitating (Crane, 1999: 73–8). British researchers (Timms and Fry, 1989) studied a group with mental health problems living in a Salvation Army hostel in southeast London. Here the researchers found that in all cases mental health difficulties had preceded the loss of accommodation (Timms, 1993: 99). In a study of nearly 700 homeless individuals with mental health problems in the United States, Sullivan et al. (2000: 448) found that about two thirds had became homeless after the onset of their illness and this group was more likely to suffer from schizophrenia or bipolar disorder. The connection between schizophrenia and long-term intractable homelessness has also been noted in other studies (Weller, 1986; Olfson et al., 1999).

Many studies find little or no connection between discharge from a psychiatric hospital and immediate homelessness (Crane, 1999; Cleary and Prizeman, 1998). However, the loss of many psychiatric beds has meant that those being treated for mental illness that cannot live at home may be referred into settings that cannot address their mental health needs. The Irish Simon Community noted that:

> emergency hostels and shelters do not provide 'therapeutic communities' and with their large transitory populations, they are simply unsuitable for people with psychiatric problems. Yet such hostels . . . appear to be a major accommodation referral option for the psychiatric services
>
> (Collins and McKeown, 1992: 35)

Similarly bed & breakfast accommodation, used widely in Ireland to house the homeless, is also unsuitable and Focus Ireland have highlighted its inappropriateness in terms of privacy and social isolation and its impact on the physical and emotional health of the homeless population who use it (Houghton and Hickey, 2000: 6). Certainly what emerges from these and other studies is that individuals with vulnerable mental health may enter a state of homelessness as a result of significant crises in their lives for which they are ill prepared to cope. The impact of being homeless or of being sheltered in emergency accommodation only adds to pre-existing mental anguish. Fernandez (1996: 225) stresses that access to day facilities and a range of well-structured ancillary mental health services is required for the majority of such individuals.

Mental health difficulties caused by homelessness

Even without a pre-existing mental health difficulty, living on the streets or in hostel accommodation causes a decline in self-esteem and leads to depression and feelings of helplessness and hopelessness (Snow and Anderson, 1993; Rosenthal, 1994; Feeney et al., 2000; Downer, 2001). In a large American study, Sullivan et al. (2000) found that approximately one third of the homeless mentally ill became homeless prior to the onset of mental health difficulties. This was an ethnically diverse group with poor levels of education who were more likely to suffer from depression than from schizophrenia or bipolar disorder. This was also a group with the highest levels of childhood poverty and physical abuse and almost one third had been homeless as children. Sullivan et al. (2000: 448) noted that these were individuals marked by extreme disadvantage, where homelessness in adulthood was a continuation of earlier disruptive and deprived conditions.

Psychological distress that comes as a direct consequence of homelessness can also lead on to a deterioration in the already highly stressful state of being out-of-home. In her work on homelessness among mothers with children, Downer (2001: 10–11) noted that feelings of depression, fear, anger and anxiety engendered by homelessness produced negative self-perceptions among mothers and negative parent–child relationships. Similarly the depression brought about by homelessness can immobilise people, thus severely limiting their ability to find new accommodation or to accept help from appropriate services (Crane, 1999).

Alcohol and drug misuse

It is estimated that the rate of alcohol misuse in homeless people is three to five times higher than that of the general population (Williams and Avebury, 1995: 28–9). The misuse of alcohol and/or drugs by many homeless may pre-date and be one of the causes of their homelessness. For others, alcohol and drug misuse may have been adopted or increased as a way of coping with homelessness. Balazs's work in the East End of London found that heavy drinking had damaging effects on both physical and mental health including minor degrees of brain damage. Balazs also found that prescribed medication to alleviate depression could become of source of drug addiction (1993: 78–9). A study of the health of the homeless population in Dublin found a very high level of alcohol use, especially among men, with one in four in the study suffering from alcoholism (Condon, 2001: 32). This study confirmed that smoking, alcohol abuse and illicit drug use were very common amongst homeless people with very serious results for both their physical and mental health (Condon, 2001: 64). Other recent Irish studies show similar figures for alcohol abuse with between one third and one half of those who are homeless drinking heavily or very heavily (Holohan, 1997; Cleary and Prizeman, 1998; Feeney et al., 2000). Illicit drug abuse among the homeless population is also growing. O'Gorman (2002), in her review of the Irish situation, reported that contemporary studies put the figure for drug abuse in the Irish homeless population somewhere between 24 and 41 per cent. However, she cautions that the true figure for drug misuse in Ireland may be higher than this and there is evidence that there are high levels of drug-related risk behaviour, particularly in the younger age group (2002: 9).

The above discussion should not imply that all homeless people who abuse drugs and/or alcohol are, by default, mentally ill. However, heavy drug and alcohol abuse has a significantly damaging effect on the physical and psychological health of those who are homeless (Koegel and Burnam, 1988). Drake et al. put the figure for those with a dual diagnosis of severe mental illness and substance abuse at about 10–20 per cent of the homeless population (1991: 1149) and Breaky's research found it to be 24 per cent (1996: 115).

For those with a dual diagnosis of mental illness and alcohol/substance abuse, treatment and support can be very complicated. The Irish Homeless Agency (Homeless Agency, 2004: 51) notes that in 2001 homeless people with high support needs who had drug or alcohol problems or exhibited challenging behaviour were excluded from most services and forced to sleep rough. In the Irish context, Crowley (2003) also observes that homeless people with a dual diagnosis of mental illness and drug misuse often find themselves without a service as 'existing services consider themselves to be either psychiatric services or addiction services with poorly defined collaborative functions (Crowley, 2003: 28). Many studies (Hopper, 1989; Drake et al., 1989) advocate an integrated service approach to this group. This is one which is less focused on treatment and more on the provision of basic services, most notably housing, 'for those with alcohol and drug problems, including those dually diagnosed, maintaining sobriety may be impossible practically without adequate housing' (Drake et al., 1989: 1155). This then becomes more about creating supportive environments for these most vulnerable individuals than instituting treatment programmes (Koegel and Burnam, 1988). *Homelessness: An Integrated Strategy* (Department of the Environment and Local Government, 2000: 38) noted that funding had been provided by the government for the establishment in the Dublin area of two high support specialist hostels for homeless persons with drug and alcohol addictions to minimise harming themselves and to provide a suitable platform for access to essential treatment.

Children and young people

the consequences of homelessness on children are dire. Homelessness robs children during their critical formative years of the basic resources needed for normal development . . . they undergo events that contribute to medical, emotional and behavioural problems that may be of lasting duration.

(Downer, 2001: 17)

The UN Committee on the Rights of the Child in a report on Ireland expressed particular concern about the incidence of child poverty and homeless children in the State (Children's Rights Alliance, 1998: 8). The Committee also commented on the lack of adequate programmes and services addressing the mental health of children and their families. In the homeless population, there are two separate categories of children: those who are part of homeless families with one or both parents, and those older homeless children and adolescents who are alone. However, in many cases, a young person may graduate from the first to the second group and studies have shown that children in homeless families have a high risk for poor physical and mental health (Bassuk, 1984; Collins and McKeown, 1992). The literature suggests that most homeless families are single parent families, in most cases headed by a mother (Halpenny et al., 2001). The impact of homelessness and the almost inevitable poverty that accompanies it can have a severe effect on the mental health of women trying to parent alone with nowhere to live. Research also shows that many homeless mothers suffer from depression (Cumella et al., 1998; Lang et al., 1996) and that the low esteem experienced by many homeless mothers can have a seriously detrimental effect on their ability to parent effectively (Boxhill and Beaty, 1987; Downer, 2001). In addition, many homeless families may also have entered the homeless state from situations of family breakdown, violence or substance abuse. Irish studies indicate that many of the women entering homelessness had been in care at some point and/or had been exposed to violence and sexual abuse (Halpenny et al., 2001: 5).

Children as part of homeless families
The impact of living in a homeless family can have a profound impact on children. In a study in the United States, Bassuk (1984) found that most of the children living with their families in a homeless shelter showed high levels of anxiety, severe depression and half needed psychiatric evaluation. In an Irish

pilot study of homeless children living with their families, Focus Ireland found that the life stress scale scores for 71 per cent of the mothers were critically high. They also found that half of the children exhibited symptoms that indicated they had mental health problems of sufficient severity to merit referral for psychiatric assessment (Focus Ireland et al., 2000: 21–3). Likewise Halpenny et al. found that many parents living in emergency accommodation were concerned about the effects of homelessness on the mental health of their children in terms of anxiety, depression and isolation (2001: 51). For many homeless families in Ireland, the policy response has been to place them in emergency accommodation, in either bed and breakfast or hostel settings. They pointed out that such placements made it difficult or impossible for children to develop normal family routines as children are often confined to one room or forced to leave their accommodation for periods during the day (2001). This can adversely affect interaction with parents and siblings thus increasing behavioural difficulties and strained family relationships. Criticism of the over use in Ireland of emergency settings, particularly bed and breakfast accommodation has been widespread. Focus Ireland's Annual Report for 2003 argued that the average time many families with children spend living in emergency bed and breakfast accommodation has grown from 20 days in 1993 to an average time of 18 months in 2004. The Homeless Agency's action plan on homelessness in Dublin 2004–6 (Homeless Agency, 2004) has proposed a new project where fifty homeless people, selected randomly, will be placed directly into rented housing rather than emergency accommodation. This approach has a number of potential benefits, including the immediate integration of those households, and cost savings. Tenancies would be 'conditional on compliance with a support programme, if necessary, provided on an outreach basis' (Homeless Agency, 2004: 14). The reality is that even if this initiative is successful, it will be too late for many young children who may be irrovocably damaged by their experiences of being on the street or in short-term accommodation.

Young single homeless
The figures for young people (aged under 18 years) who are out of home have been growing both nationally and internationally (Bhugra, 1996; Vostanis et al., 1998; Kellegher et al., 2000). Focus Ireland has seen the numbers increase substantially to the point where 13 per cent of the homeless people seeking services from their Outreach Team were under 18 years of age (Focus Ireland, undated: 71). Focus Ireland also identified that significant numbers of young people leaving state care were becoming homeless, with 68 per cent of those who left health board care experiencing homelessness within two years (Kellegher et al., 2000: 15). Other Irish studies have highlighted the unsuitable use of Garda [police] stations and children's hospitals as accommodation for homeless young people (Youth Homelessness Strategy, 2001). Furthermore, drug abuse,

alcohol abuse, prostitution, psychiatric and psychological difficulties have all been identified as problems associated with youth homelessness (Department of Health and Children, 2001g). The Report of the Forum on Youth Homelessness (Northern Area Health Board, 2000) noted that many young people who were out of home displayed disturbed or difficult behaviour such as self-harm, aggression and violence and that such behaviour further isolated them from services. The report went on to identify that mental health services provided for this group of young people were difficult to access and, in many cases, were unsuitable for their needs. In line with other research, the report acknowledged that emergency accommodation offered to young people with mental health difficulties was inappropriate for their needs and likely to exacerbate their illness (2000: 47–9).

The last few years have seen the publication of a number of important policy and legislative publications in relation to Irish youth homelessness. Section 5 of the Irish 1991 Childcare Act had placed a legal obligation on health boards to meet the accommodation and other needs of homeless children, that is those under the age of 18. Subsequent to this, the National Children's Strategy (Department of Health and Children, 2000a) identified the development of a National Youth Homelessness Strategy as a priority in addressing Irish youth homelessness. The Strategy reported in 2001 with the goal

> to reduce and if possible eliminate youth homelessness through preventative strategies and where a child becomes homeless to ensure that he/she benefits from a comprehensive range of services aimed at reintegrating him/her into his/her community as quickly as possible.
>
> (Department of Health and Children, 2001g: 3)

Around the same time, the Forum on Youth Homelessness was established to draw up a plan to improve and develop services for young homeless people in the Eastern Health Board area; the Forum's report was published in 2000. These publications have continued to highlight the difficulties of inadequate and patchy service provision and have stressed the need for services for young homeless people to be made more comprehensive and co-ordinated. They have also acknowledged the vulnerability of children leaving state care to homelessness and poor mental health as identified by Focus Ireland (Kellegher et al., 2000). The Youth Homelessness Strategy proposes the establishment of comprehensive aftercare plans for young people leaving care and have suggested the provision of key workers to co-ordinate the specific needs of young people either homeless or at risk of homelessness.

Amnesty International (Crowley, 2003: 32) has expressed concern that Ireland does not comply with its international obligations under the UN Convention on the Rights of the Child, in its treatment of homeless children with, or at risk of, mental illness. Certainly, until the recommendations outlined in the Youth Homeless Strategy (Department of Health and Children, 2001g) are implemented as a matter of urgency, we are in danger of raising another generation of young people on the streets in situations of misery and degradation. Not only this but, as so much of the research points out, they are highly likely to grow into homeless adults with significant and intractable mental health difficulties.

Women and homelessness

For many years there was an assumption that most if not all homeless people were male, typified by the lone male street drinker and many earlier studies and some recent ones have focused on this latter population. In Ireland, the work of Sister Stanilaus Kennedy in the mid-1980s highlighted the needs of homeless women in Dublin to whom she referred as 'the hidden homeless' (Kennedy, 1985). Kennedy's research revealed these women to be poorly educated, unskilled and caught in a cycle of homelessness. Many had left home as a result of family violence and incest. Of the women she interviewed in long-term hostels, 31 per cent had intellectual disability, 22 per cent had mental health problems and 14 per cent suffered from alcoholism (Kennedy, 1985: 132). This study proved the catalyst for the setting up of the Focus Ireland services for homeless people.

Women are still in the minority in the homeless population, with 81 per cent of the single homeless adults in the Dublin area in 2002 being male (Williams and Gorby, 2002). The same study noted that the majority of homeless families were single parent units, 81 per cent of which were those of lone mothers. These figures are similar to international data on homeless women, with many women concealing their homelessness for as long as possible by staying with friends or remaining in unsatisfactory or potentially violent relationships (Marshall, 1996: 64; Smith, 1999). Research from both Britain and the United States shows that lone, homeless women tend to be younger than their male counterparts. They are also more likely to have remained in education, to have held a job, to have contact with friends and to have been married with children at some stage of their lives (Digby, 1976; Drake et al., 1982; Breaky et al., 1989; Marshall, 1996). International studies also indicate that there is an over-representation of ethnic minorities in the population of homeless women. Data for homelessness in Dublin in 2002 showed that ten per cent of homeless lone parents (81 per cent of whom are lone mothers) were born outside Ireland (Williams and Gorby, 2002).

The previous section on children and young people has already discussed how attempting to raise children while homeless puts considerable stress on the mental health of mothers. Studies also indicate that many homeless women have experienced violence throughout their lifetime from childhood abuse to violence from spouses or partners (Bassuk et al., 1998; Browne, 1993). On the whole, homeless mothers report higher levels of stress, depression, and poorer coping strategies than low-income, housed mothers (Banyard and Graham-Bermann, 1998). An Irish study (Smith et al., 2001) also found that drug abuse was a feature in the lives of homeless mothers, the majority of whom had sought or were taking drug treatment.

The pattern of mental health for lone, homeless women differs from that of homeless mothers, and studies show that lone, homeless women have high rates of schizophrenia (Marshall, 1996: 75). Bassuk at al. (1986) found that in a group of 80 homeless mothers, those without children had the highest rates for schizophrenia, generalised anxiety disorder and alcohol abuse; 72 per cent of this group had a lifetime psychiatric diagnosis. Balazs (1993) also found that the prevalence of severe mental health problems in lone, homeless women was three times higher than in homeless men. He argued the reason for this might be because family and friends could offer accommodation to a woman for longer periods of time than they could a man, therefore lone women who become homeless may have chronic and intractable mental illness (1993: 71). Marshall (1996: 73) differentiates between the life patterns of younger homeless mothers (mostly parenting children) and single, older homeless women using different models of homelessness. The 'periodic/cyclical' model is one where women are intermittently homeless, with younger mothers being more likely to experience this type of homelessness. Older single women are most likely to enter homelessness through the 'slip/slide' model where they experience a combination of several events leading to a downward spiral. With these older single women, episodes of severe mental illness are likely to characterise this decline into homelessness.

National and international policy reports indicate that the services for homeless women are poor and there is a dearth of plans for the specific needs of women with mental health difficulties. In their work on homelessness at European level, Edgar and Doherty (2001) note that the needs of many homeless women in Europe are inadequately or inappropriately provided for by existing homeless services. Referring to reports from the European Observatory on Homelessness, they suggest that the provision of social protection for women exposed to the risk of homelessness is patchy, with services for lone parents being more developed than services for older women or those women who are victims of domestic violence (2001: 17). O'Sullivan and Higgins argue that up to the late 1970s, the familialistic nature of the Irish welfare state rendered homelessness among women as a hidden phenomenon. Even with recent changes in Irish welfare, the visibility of Irish homeless women remains low (2001: 88). The 2000 report of the Department of the Environment and Local Government, *Homelessness: An Integrated Strategy*, records that the housing provision for homeless women is inadequate with fewer than 100 hostel places available for women in Dublin and an estimated one third of these occupied on a long-term basis. Specific plans by the Homeless Agency for services to homeless women in the period 2004–6 is confined to a proposal for six units of housing for women and children fleeing domestic violence.

Flexible services to meet challenging needs

Harvey notes that, compared with other European countries, services for the homeless in Ireland rely disproportionately on voluntary organisations (1998: 9). In the past, Irish voluntary service providers, such as Trust and the Simon Community, have provided a limited but indispensable service to the homeless mentally ill, primarily caring for their basic physical needs on the street or in 'drop-in' centres. Focus Ireland also provided some of the first units of supported accommodation where vulnerable tenants received the long-term help and support of a key worker, a practice now offered by number of other social housing agencies. However, such services cannot fully meet the complex needs of the homeless mentally ill without the back-up of comprehensive mental health supports. A major requirement in the provision of such services must be a move away from catchment-based psychiatric services where an individual is required to attend the psychiatric services in the area in which he or she lives. As Brooke (2002: 15) points out, this is a real Catch 22, where if you are homeless you cannot live in a catchment area, if you do not live in a catchment area you cannot access services. McKeown (1999: 19) also considers the need for services to become flexible and removed from a catchment area basis. He argues that this approach should be central to a new strategic vision for mental health services for the homeless.

For many years, the only state specialist psychiatric service caring specifically for the homeless was that based in St Brendan's Hospital in Dublin. Called the Programme for the Homeless, it was founded in 1979 by Dr Joe Fernandez to offer psychiatric residential care, including acute beds, for homeless people with mental health problems and day support services, including nursing cover and a follow-up service into the community (Fernandez, 1996: 222). Now based in a city-centre location, the programme provides food, financial management, washing facilities and medical attention, including medication. The service has also set up three community houses that provide varying degrees of support (Brooke, 2002: 18).

The impact of more recent policy initiatives has resulted in the development of similar, flexible services. *Homelessness: An Integrated Strategy* (Department of the Environment and Local Government, 2000) required health boards to put in place a range of service provisions to meet the health needs of homeless people and the 2002 *Homeless Preventative Strategy* (Department of the Environment and Local Government) has obligated health boards to put protocols in place for those being discharged from acute and psychiatric hospitals. In 2004 two new multi-disciplinary primary care teams were set up, one in Dublin and one in Cork. In addition, two primary care units have been established in Dublin-based inner city homeless services. The Homeless Agency, operating on a basis of partnership and inter-agency collaboration, is also committed to ensuring that homeless people have access to a full range of health board services, including those targeted at mental health. Although these developments give some cause for optimism, it will take a number of years to see if the quality and scale of these new initiatives are enough to meet the needs of a group who have been marginalised for a very long time. Most urgently required are appropriate and flexible mental health services for those who are homeless and who have mental health difficulties. The first report of the Inspector of Mental Health Services (Carey, 2004: 33) noted that homeless people tended to encounter mental health services in situations of acute social stress and, not infrequently, with acute psychosis. The Inspector recommended the provision of specialist services to meet these specific needs. The Mental Health Commission's Strategic Plan for 2004–5 notes that one of the challenges facing them includes addressing the gaps and deficiencies in services for homeless people with mental illness, yet no specific recommendations are offered in the plan as to how this may be advanced (Mental Health Commission, 2004c).

In simple terms, the homeless mentally ill do not easily fit into the policy solutions for the majority of those who are homeless and, certainly, the provision of extra independent housing in itself is unlikely to address their complex needs. While recent and Irish policy changes look potentially promising, the figures of those who are homeless and in need of mental health services in Ireland continue to grow (O'Brien, 2005). It is evident that no single reason emerges for people becoming homeless with attendant poor mental health; rather it is the result of a combination of factors, most of which are foreseeable and open to remedial action. Thus, the complex and challenging needs of those who are homeless with mental health problems require policy responses that are based in concrete undertaking rather than, as Amnesty describes current Irish policies, 'too aspirational to guarantee effectiveness' (2003: 48).

> [I]n proposing a strategy for meeting the needs of people who are mentally ill and homeless, it needs to be acknowledged that the present system does not work and is fundamentally at odds with equity, quality of service and accountability which are at the core of health care policy in Ireland.
>
> (McKeown, 1999: 23)

Chapter 13

Mental health and Ireland's new communities

Joe Moran

Historical overview

The number of immigrants who have come to live in Ireland in recent years has been relatively small when compared to the mass emigration from Ireland that took place from the early part of the nineteenth century. It was not until as recently as the 1990s that Ireland's haemorrhage of people began to slow down and people from other countries regarded Ireland as a place to which they might migrate. Ireland has in this short period become a country of net immigration (see figure 13.1).

Figure 13.1 **Population and migration estimates**

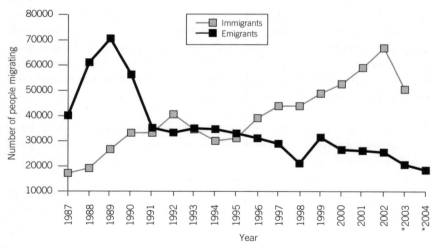

Source: CSO, Sept. 2004

This reversal was as a result of a new partnership model of corporate economic planning begun in 1987. The partnership model was laid on the joint foundation stones of large financial transfers from the European Union and years of investment in education. The growth in employment in the 1990s was reflected in a falling unemployment rate and an increase in the number of women who joined the paid workforce. From the mid-1990s onwards there is a correlation between growth in employment and increased immigration, to a point where Ireland is only second to Luxembourg in the EU in the level of annual immigration (Immigrant Council of Ireland, 2003).

While much of this immigration consists of returned Irish emigrants, as well as people from the United Kingdom, other European Union countries, North America and Australia, there has been a substantial growth in the number of people who have come to Ireland as migrant workers, students and asylum seekers from Central and Eastern Europe, Africa and Asia. Between the Irish censuses of 1996 and 2002 the numbers of people who were born in these three areas of the world increased from 16,622 to 78,882. The growth in the number of immigrants reached an historic high of 66,900 in the twelve months to April 2002 and fell back to 50,100 in the twelve-month period to April 2004 (CSO, 2004). Among these figures the number of asylum applicants fell back from 11,634 in 2002 to 7,900 in 2003 and 3,132 at the end of August 2004 (Office of the Refugee Applications Commissioner, 2004). The Immigrant Council of Ireland (2003) questions the reliability of the figures used in counting immigrants. In a study by the Immigrant Council of Ireland (2003) it is suggested that these figures are an underestimation and that the number of immigrants in Ireland is in fact greater than official sources indicate.

Whatever the exact numbers of immigrants in Ireland, it is evident that for the first time Ireland has a diverse population which is growing. This diversity poses challenges for social policy makers across a range of policy areas including that of mental health. The mental health of Ireland's new communities is an area which to date has received little attention in policy or practice, but it is an important one for policy makers and practitioners alike. It is also potentially a hugely controversial area as the nature of the debate about mental well-being and mental ill-health, difficult even among a generally mono-cultural popu-lation, becomes more contentious when one begins to consider the mental health needs of people from diverse populations.

The international context

There are a number of international instruments and principles which directly address mental health issues and a number of others that are relevant to persons with a mental illness. Similarly there are also international instruments and principles that deal with or allude to the rights of immigrants. Relevant instruments include:

- Universal Declaration of Human Rights
- European Convention for the Protection of Human Rights
- International Covenant on Civil and Political Rights
- International Covenant on Economic, Social and Cultural Rights
- Council of Europe Recommendation Concerning the Legal Protection of Persons Suffering from Mental Disorders
- International Convention on the Protection of the Rights of All Migrant Workers and Members of Their Families
- Geneva Convention Relating to the Status of Refugees
- UN Principles for the Protection of Persons with Mental Illness and the Improvement of Mental Care

These international instruments offer some comfort to immigrants in their general assertions on fundamental rights, the provision of equality of treatment with nationals, and the provision of treatment which does not discriminate against them. However, there is no guarantee that states will adhere to their obligations under these international instruments. In reporting to the Economic and Social Council the UN High Commissioner for Human Rights stated:

> Persons with functional limitation or disabilities are particularly vulnerable to exclusion and marginalisation. Because of their physical or mental limitations, persons with disabilities are frequently more at risk of having their rights violated and denied. (UN High Commissioner for Human Rights, 2001: para 48)

In this reference, the High Commissioner was referring to the general population and not to immigrants. The potential for persons who are immigrants to have their rights violated and denied are even greater than for nationals as there are few specific detailed obligations to take into account the needs of immigrants in these international instruments. There are some implicit references to the difficulties immigrants may face in their use or contacts with mental health services. For example, the European Convention for the Protection of Human Rights refers to informing those detained 'in a language which he understands' (Article 5.2). The UN Principles for the Protection of Persons with Mental Illness and the Improvement of Mental Health Care (the MI Principles) includes in its principles those who may not be speakers of the native tongue(s) of a state or be of the same cultural background as the majority population. Principle 7.3 states that 'every patient shall have the right to treatment suited to his or her cultural background'. On the issue of consent Principle 11.2 states that 'informed consent is consent obtained freely, without threats or improper inducements, after appropriate disclosure to the patient of adequate and under-standable information in a form and language understood by the patient'. Likewise, on the issue of notice of rights, the MI Principles also require patients to be informed in a language and form which they understand. The MI Principles refer to one other issue of relevance to those who may not have the language of the country in which she or he seeks mental health services. Principle 18 states that 'the patient shall also be entitled to the assistance, if necessary, of the services of an interpreter'.

In a number of respects these international instruments are vague and appear limited in their application for immigrants, as it remains the responsi-bility of the country in which they are living to provide services in accordance with their own policy-making priorities and financial resources. Yet they do provide the basis for increased protection and assistance for immigrants if the states in which they live are party to international conventions which may relate to them. States that are party to international conventions are periodically called to account for their policies in relation to these conventions. Such accountability offers some comfort to immigrants in relation to mental health and many other social, political, economic and civil rights.

Current policy

There are no national policies in place for the mental health of new communities in Ireland. People from new communities who wish to use mental health services must do so on the same basis as Irish nationals. While there are no national poli-cies in place there are two services which meet in part the mental health needs of sections of our new communities. The Refugee Psychological Service provided through the Northern Area Health Board is based in Dublin and located at St Brendan's Hospital; and the Centre for the Care of Survivors of Torture which has been developed by the non-governmental organisation SPIRASI, also based in Dublin and geographically very close to St Brendan's Hospital.

The Refugee Psychological Service was originally established during the Bosnian refugee programme in 1993 to provide psychological support for the Bosnian programme refugees who had been invited to Ireland by the Irish gov-ernment. This service was expanded in 1999 and subsequently, to provide a service for Kosovar programme refugees and the increasing numbers of asylum seekers entering the country. The service also provides a dedicated clinical psychologist for unaccompanied asylum seeking children and young people. The service provides short-term intervention for newly arrived asylum seekers who are accommodated in one of three reception centres in Dublin (Clarke, 2001). The Centre for the Care and Survivors of Torture was established in 2001. This non-governmental organisation provides, as its name suggests, a service to the survivors of torture. The service includes counselling, the documenting of torture, and writing medico-legal reports for asylum seekers in the asylum process (O'Sullivan 2002). Both of these services contribute to the mental well being and treatment of some of the most vulnerable people in Ireland's new communities. However, because of their Dublin location and the composition of their client groups, both of these services meet only some of the mental health needs of people from new communities.

There are no data available on the extent of the usage of psychiatric services by immigrants in Ireland. On the other hand, what we do know of the mental health services in Ireland means it is unlikely that they are well placed to deal with people from new communities. Mental health policy in Ireland has been described by one commentator as 'backwards into the future' (Powell, 1998). A number of reports published during 2003–4 have been critical of the mental health services in Ireland. O'Keane et al. (2003) highlight the inequitable distribution of mental health services throughout the country, demonstrating that the most affluent areas have the greatest psychiatric resources. Furthermore, they say that mental health services are overstretched and their availability is limited. O'Keane et al. (2003) were especially critical of the lack of availability of specialist services and that apart from basic specialist services for older people and children, specialist services were not found outside Dublin. They claim that the development of mental health services in Ireland has taken place without considering socio-political or demographic realities and they suggest a number of reasons for the existence of such problems. These include underfunding of the mental health services over a long period of time, a high level of temporary consultant contracts, and the lack of a national mental health strategy (O'Keane et al., 2003).

A second report published in 2003 by Amnesty International was a review of how the rights of people with mental illness are respected in Ireland. The Amnesty report was critical of mental health policy in a number of ways: underresourcing; poor services planning; and that the Mental Health Act 2001 does not reflect the full range of international human rights standards. Among the recommendations of the Amnesty report was that specialised mental health care should be provided for all who need it including asylum seekers, refugees and other minority groups (Amnesty International, 2003).

In the final Report of the Inspector of Mental Hospitals 2003, whose function has been assumed by the newly established Mental Health Commission from January 2004, the Inspectorate acknowledged that progress has taken place since 1987 (when it began its work) in the provision of mental health services. However, many deficits remain in the provision of mental health services throughout the state. The Inspectorate points out that there are problems in terms of equity and fairness within the provision of services, and that the majority of services operated 'partially developed conservative community models' (Department of Health and Children, 2004b: 2). On the issue of funding, the Inspectorate does not accept the 'under-funding' argument as it is normally advanced. However, the Inspectorate does question the efficiency of expenditure in this area and states that 'there are considerable disparities, which are historical rather than based on any rational or epidemiological considerations' (2004: 5). It is apparent from the Report that groups with special needs within Irish society fare badly, such as the intellectually disabled, the homeless mentally ill, and children and adolescents.

The challenges of mental health provision for Ireland's new communities

While there are very obvious challenges facing the state in the provision of mental health services in general, there have been some important policy commitments which in time should improve these services. The National Health Strategy *Quality and Fairness: A Health System for You* (Department of Health and Children, 2001b) gave a commitment to ensuring quality and high standards in the delivery of mental health services by agreeing to prepare a new National Policy Framework for the further modernisation of the mental health services in Ireland. There is an admission in the strategy that existing services are inadequate in their general provision and for specific groups. The strategy names a number of groups that are provided with inadequate services but does not include people from new communities (2001b). In a subsequent document, *Action Plan for People Management in the Health Services*, there was an acknow-ledgement of increasing numbers of non-Irish staff in the workforce and amongst the users of services, which it stated had implications for managing diversity (Department of Health and Children, 2002). Although there is a lack of recognition of the needs of people from new communities in the proposals in the National Health Strategy, the commitment to improve mental health services for the population generally is an important step. For without a general improvement in the mental health services in Ireland the chances of the mental health needs of ethnic minorities being addressed would be less likely.

In developing mental health policy for Ireland's new communities there are a number of important and challenging issues which need to be considered to ensure the delivery of quality services for these groups. The following are two of the most important issues:

- migration and mental health
- racism, culture and mental health.

Migration and mental health

Migration, planned and forced, has had a long history throughout the world. It is normally a complex act derived from a potential myriad of reasons for choosing such a path (Smaje, 1996). There are push and pull factors, personal, economic, social and political reasons for leaving one's own country and moving to another. Whatever the reasons, migration usually brings with it stress that has not been encountered before. Sluzki (1979 cited in Woodcock, 1995) argues that migration is inherently stressful. The act of emigrating from one's own country poses a major challenge to the individual and his or her family. Even those who have spent a great amount of time planning and researching their move to another country cannot prepare themselves for the shock such a move might bring. As a result the period of adjustment may take many years, if it is ever complete.

Smaje (1996) suggests that a number of factors influence the mental health of migrants. High expectations achieved or dashed may have a traumatic effect on a migrant who has moved in order to make a new life. Economic motives for migrating may lead to racialised patterns of living in a new country when the immigrant finds him or herself moving to an area where others from the same country of origin or other immigrants reside. Low pay for immigrants may lead to poor health (mental and physical) outcomes not just for the original immigrant but for generations of his or her family into the future. The immigrant may be better off financially in the host society than she or he was in their own country but in comparison to nationals they may be at an economic and social disadvantage. The effect of low levels of income, poor housing and unemployment make immigrants more susceptible to poor health. There may also be an impact on the lifestyle, social networks and kinship of the immigrant. Smaje (1996) also points out that racism directly impacts on victims through stress, injury and death, and indirectly through discrimination in the labour and housing markets.

Many groups of immigrants may be isolated in their host countries. Lam et al. (1995), in reference to Chinese families in Britain, state that they 'can be remarkably isolated from the local community or culture as a whole. This partly reflects the fact that parents have to struggle hard to establish themselves here' (1995: 283). Lam et al. (1995) say that long working hours provide little opportunity for these immigrants to find out more about the host community and they may also have a poor command of English. It is certain that it is not just the Chinese in Britain who have experienced isolation in their host countries. Many other immigrant groups have found themselves similarly isolated, including the Irish in Britain, although not necessarily for the same reasons (Pilgrim and Rogers, 1999).

Cultural expectations and norms are often seriously questioned in the new society, which may lead to fractures in relationships. These difficulties can occur between spouses, between parents and children, and between grandparents and their grandchildren. Sluzki (1979) suggests that polarisations inevitably occur within families, for instance, between those who plan for the future and those who hold on to the past. Thai (2002) outlines in a case study the polarisation between a Vietnamese immigrant couple in the United States, the man holding on to the traditional male patriarchal role of his country of origin and the woman seeking equality in her relationship with him as she had come to expect in her host society.

Asylum seekers and refugees, by the nature of forced exile, are more likely to be confronted with greater experiences of personal and social upheaval than economic migrants. Finlay and Reynolds (1987) describe the accumulation of losses suffered by asylum seekers and refugees as 'a process of bereavement' (Finlay and Reynolds, 1987: 96). As a result refugees and asylum seekers are more likely than the rest of the population to face mental health difficulties (Clarke, 2001). In a review of the research evidence of psychiatric morbidity in refugee populations, Ramsay and Gorst-Unsworth (2003) found that there are variations in rates of morbidity, in particular in the factors related with the trauma which led to exile and the factors connected with the exile experience. The evidence suggests that trauma experienced pre-exile, and subsequent social experiences in exile, constitute independent factors. The severity of the reaction to these events and any consequent psychiatric morbidity depend on many variables from the extent of trauma experienced, the proximity to trauma, threat to life, personality factors, affective social supports, delays in processing asylum applications, detention, the reception in the host country, unemployment and poverty (Ramsay and Gorst-Unsworth, 2003). It is clearly evident from their review of the research literature that refugees constitute a population at risk from mental disorder. Yet, according to Watters (1998), it is important to distinguish between distress and clinically defined mental illness. He makes the point that mental health professionals should be careful about how they apply Western definitions of psychological ill-health to refugees as it may not always be appropriate or helpful. Summerfield (1996) questions the 'traumatisation' of the ordinary distress and suffering of war by Western mental health experts, which he describes as a pseudo-condition for the vast majority of those caught up in such events. He says that this narrow approach may create inappropriate sick roles and sidelines the proper incorporation of people's own capacities into strategies for their creative survival.

Racism, culture and mental health
The challenge for mental health professionals of understanding the impact of the migration process on people from new communities and the consequences for their mental health is surpassed by the challenge of understanding their work in the contexts of culture and racism. Racism, culture and mental health

have long been debated in other countries where a substantial critical literature has been developed. This literature covers a range of crucial issues relevant to the practice of psychiatry with people from ethnic minority groups, including the response of psychiatry to their mental health needs, the appropriateness of the mental health models used in treatment, and the issue of racism.

The relationship between psychiatry, and health models generally, and ethnic minorities in many Western countries is based on the assumption that individual, family and community problems are somehow 'internally generated' (Stubbs, 1993: 40). In other words, families from ethnic minorities are pathologised and generalised traits are used to inform the views of white professional practice (Stubbs 1993; Pilgrim and Rogers, 1999). A typical example of this approach is towards the Asian community in Britain. Watters (1996) deconstructs the representations of the mental health of Asians in British psychiatry in which he challenges the assumptions and stereotypes of particular views of Asian people's problems which in turn impact on the mental health services this community receives.

As a result of these assumptions, mental health services provided to ethnic minorities in multi-ethnic societies have been criticised for focusing 'on what has been perceived to be differential assessment' (Solomon, 2001: 190). Solomon continues:

> Reports from several countries indicate that ethnic minorities are more likely to be diagnosed as suffering from psychosis, be admitted involuntarily to hospitals, remain for longer periods in the hospital and be treated with medication rather than by counselling or social rehabilitation' (Solomon, 2001: 190).

Some commentators regard the approach to ethnic minorities in psychiatry as part of a more general societal method of social control (Stubbs, 1993). Pilgrim and Rogers (1999) suggest that psychiatry for ethnic minorities is concerned with 'the segregation or exclusion of threatening or undesirable "others"' (Pilgrim and Rogers, 1999: 81). Psychiatry is therefore regarded as part of the state's repressive apparatus to discourage immigration, and as a practice is perceived to be coercive.

The appropriateness of mental health models used to meet the needs of ethnic minorities is usually contextualised within the term 'culture'. The most frequent response to meeting the needs of ethnic minorities in the provision of mental health services is therefore to improve the cultural understanding of the professionals who provide these services. This takes the form of 'ethnic sensitivity', which according to Stubbs (1993) has been institutionalised in the provision of welfare services in the United Kingdom. He points to a number of characteristics of ethnic sensitivity but highlights the existence of different cultural patterns among immigrants as being the most emphasised. This is underpinned by an ideology of 'multi-culturalism'. He states that: 'In terms of service delivery, the argument is that there needs to be a better understanding of such things as the customs, traditions and religious activities of ethnic minority groups' (Stubbs 1993: 38).

Despite the fact that the ethnic sensitivity approach has been in existence for many years, the culturally different are still viewed as 'exotic' which means foreign or different or deviant (Acharyya, 1996). The problem with the use of 'culture' as the term of reference is that it leads to stereotypes rather than providing for a flexible source for living. Instead it is 'a rigid and constraining concept which is seen somehow to mechanistically determine peoples' behaviours and actions' (Ahmad, 1996:190). For a number of commentators the problem with psychiatry and ethnic minorities goes beyond culture to that of racism and structural inequalities (Ahmad, 1993; Ahmad, 1996; Fernando, 2002; Pilgrim and Rogers, 1999; Stubbs, 1993; and Turner and Kramer, 1995). There has been a strong tradition in the history of medicine of 'genetic predisposition' in some racial stocks to mental illness (Turner and Kramer, 1995). Pilgrim and Rogers (1999) state that the link between race and mental illness has been a close one, and that medical-scientific knowledge has not been neutral about this relationship. In fact they say 'it has played a significant role in the perpetuation of pejorative theories and oppressive practices about certain racial groups' (Pilgrim and Rogers, 1999: 65).

Many professionals deny that they or their practice is racist. Fernando (2002) claims that racism in psychiatry is not an aberration but the normal condition. The denial of the importance of race and culture in psychiatric practice may be termed 'the colour-blind, culture blind approach in psychiatry' (2002: 132). He claims that the colour-blind approach is defective in two ways. The first is that the professional's own racial bias is likely to be ignored or denied and therefore not taken into account. Secondly, the patient or client is invalidated by being seen as a person without colour. 'Colour represents race, an important determinant of self-perception as well as of social opportunities open to people, their rights and their experiences in a racist society' (Fernando, 2002: 132). The culture-blind approach is determined by seeing an individual without perceiving his or her culture; it also has two important defects. The first is that the person is observed outside his or her social context, outside his or her group or community. Secondly any difference observed might be perceived as an individual difference which will be judged as an aberration from the 'norm', rather than one which may reflect a cultural norm. The colour-blind, culture-blind approach in psychiatry thus falls into a trap of denying social realities of race and culture (Fernando, 2002). This denial of social realities gives rise to poor practice and a poor mental health service to people from ethnic minorities.

Likely developments and future challenges

Mental health policies and practices do not operate in a political and social vacuum. In the context of new communities and their mental health needs, mental health policies, or conversely, the lack of such policies, are influenced by wider considerations in relation to immigration. The Irish state along with the other states of the European Union has in place policies that are intended to curtail immigration. Currently Ireland has an asylum policy but it does not have an immigration policy. Ireland's asylum policy is hostile to asylum seekers, with its emphasis on control and deterrence. As a central part of its policy towards asylum seekers the state has advocated their exclusion from participation in Irish society (Fanning 2002). Ireland's short-term economic needs dictate its immigration practices, which favour the requirements of employers rather than the needs of employees. This impacts on immigrants who are from outside the European Union, as work permits are linked to the job rather than to the employee. Even for the new members of the EU differential policies have been introduced by the state.

The introduction of changes in social welfare legislation in the lead-in to the accession of ten East European and Mediterranean states acceding to the European Union in May 2004 was directly intended to deter people who did not have work from entering the state. These attitudes, practices and policy decisions impact on all aspects of state services including the provision of mental health services. These are often manifested in lesser rights and entitlements for ethnic minority groups. The decisions of the state which give lesser rights to people from new communities are described by Fanning as 'structural barriers to participation in society that compound institutional barriers resulting from racism' (Fanning, 2004: 202–3). It is therefore a challenge for those working in the mental health services to surmount the attitude of the state and provide relevant and appropriate mental health services which are inclusive rather than exclusive. The poor state of the Irish mental health services poses a major challenge to the development of inclusive services for people from new communities. In the short term it is difficult to see where the impetus for developing such services might come from. The role of the Mental Health Commission could prove pivotal, as its primary function is to 'promote and foster high standards and good practices in the delivery of mental health services' (Government of Ireland, 2001: 145).

Providing services to diverse and relatively small, if increasing, ethnic minority communities, will also be a challenge. The justification for services where there is a lack of a 'critical mass' of people in need of services will undoubtedly exercise the minds of service planners. It is most likely that without a concentration of people from ethnic minority backgrounds their needs will not even be recognised let alone planned for. There is of course the perennial issue of whether services for ethnic minorities should be part of the mainstream or whether they should be specialist. In discussing mental health services for African Americans, Turner and Kramer (1995) argue against separate service provision on the grounds that 'separatism leaves intact the social dominance of Whites; second, whenever interactions would occur – and occur they must – domination would lead to unequal distribution of resources' (1995: 15).

Expertise in this area of mental health provision in Ireland is lacking as very few professional staff from the relevant disciplines work with people from ethnic minority backgrounds. There is a need for the development of training for all in the mental health professions so that they can offer a service that meets the needs of people from ethnic minorities. One mental health professional who worked with the Refugee Psychological Service wrote candidly.

> While my training familiarised me with therapeutic approaches premised on Western cultural values I struggled with the shortcomings of such models as I attempted to employ them in addressing the needs of people from the world beyond the Western horizon. I experienced the practical and conceptual limitations of the models of therapy upon which I had previously relied far more acutely than I have when working with any other client group (Deveraux, 2000: 11).

Such training must broaden the Western knowledge base if we truly wish to respond to the mental health needs of those who come from non-Western countries. It must go beyond cultural training to include anti-racist practice and research. It is important to highlight that training which emphasises learning about culture and cultural differences may lead to reinforcing stereotypes. Moreover, it does not follow that knowledge of another's culture leads to more appropriate or effective mental health treatment (Illovsky, 2003). It is also impossible to learn about all of the different and changing cultures of the many ethnic minority groups that live in Ireland. Turner and Kramer (1995) advise 'the indispensable thing to teach is an attitude, a stance, an open-minded way of approaching the helping process with humility and a willingness to learn (Turner and Kramer, 1995: 22).

We have very little idea of what mental health problems people from the new communities have to deal with. We do not know to what extent they access mental health services or what the outcomes are for those who do. We can only guess at how appropriate or otherwise the services are for these users. Research is needed to establish some base information from which to work and to plan.

Conclusion

In truth, the mental health of new communities in Ireland has not even registered as a policy issue. It is of concern only to the small group of professional staff who work directly with or who have a personal interest in the mental health needs of Ireland's new communities, and of course for those from the new communities who need to use these services. Mental health remains a marginal issue in Irish social policy, and refugees, asylum seekers and immigrants also reside on the fringes. Add the two together and the margin increases. Nonetheless, people from these communities require and make use of mental health services. It is therefore a crucial issue for the well being of the individuals and families concerned.

We have learnt that the practice of psychiatry in other countries is controversial when it relates to ethnic minorities. Racism, culture, social control, and approaches to methods of treatment are the main elements of controversy. Addressing these issues is not easy and even in other countries, such as the UK, where immigration has a much longer history than in Ireland, there are many gaps in knowledge about the needs of particular groups of immigrants and the way forward for professional psychiatric practice is still being debated and developed (Royal College of Psychiatrists, 2003).

The development of effective policies and the provision of appropriate mental health services for Ireland's new communities are challenging. Yet the achievement of the highest standards in responding to the particular mental health needs of ethnic minorities go beyond that discipline. The provision of a mental health service that is fair, equitable and meets the highest international human rights standards reflects on how well we as the majority community treat our new communities.

References

Acharyya, S. (1996) 'Practising cultural psychiatry: the doctor's dilemma', in Heller, T., Reynolds, J., Gomm, R., Muston, R. and Pattison, S. (eds), *Mental Health Matters: A Reader.* Basingstoke: Macmillan/Open University.

Achenbach T. M., Howell C. T., McConaughy, S. H. and Stranger, C. (1995) 'Six-year predictors of problems in a national sample: III, transitions to young adult syndromes', *Journal of the American Academy of Child and Adolescent Psychiatry* 34: 658–69.

Advisory Group on Prison Deaths (1991) *Report.* Dublin: Stationery Office.

Ahmad, W. I. U. (1993) 'Making black people sick: 'race', ideology and health research', pp. 11–33 in W. I. U. Ahmad (ed.), *'Race' and Health in Contemporary Britain.* Buckingham: Open University Press.

Ahmad, W. I. U. (1996) 'The trouble with culture', in Kelleher, D. and Hillier, S. (eds), *Researching Cultural Differences in Health.* London: Routledge.

Alisky, J. M. and Iczkowski, K. A. (1990) 'Barriers to housing for deinstitutionalised psychiatric patients', *Hospital and Community Psychiatry* 41: 93–5.

Allen, M. and Cronin, J. (1992) 'Parasuicide attendances at St James Hospital Accident and Emergency Department Dublin', *Irish Social Worker* 11 (1): 13–16.

Allott, P. and Loganathan, L. (2002) *Discovering Hope for Recovery from a British Perspective: A Review Of Literature.* www.herefordshirementalhealth.info/recovery/recovery_lit

American Psychiatric Association (1994) *Diagnostic and Statistical Manual of Mental Disorders*, 4th edn. Washington DC: APA.

Amnesty International (2003) *Mental Illness: The Neglected Quarter.* Dublin, Amnesty International.

Anthony, W. (2002) 'The decade of the person and the walls that divide us' (keynote address), *Innovations in Recovery and Rehabilitation: The Decade of the Person*, 25 Oct. 2002, Boston, MA.

Appleby, L. (1985) 'Documenting the relationship between homelessness and psychiatric hospitalisation', *Hospital and Community Psychiatry* 35: 917–21.

Arboledo-Florez J. (2001) 'The state of the evidence: stigmatization and human rights violations', in *Mental Health a Call for Action by World Health Ministers.* 54th World Health Assembly Geneva: WHO.

Armstrong E. (1995) *Mental Health Issues in Primary Care: A Practical Guide.* Basingstoke: Macmillan.

Arrigo, B. A. (2001) 'Transcarceration: a constitutive ethnography of mentally ill offenders', *Prison Journal* 81 (2): 162–86.

Arthur, J. (1997) 'Psychological after-effects of abortion: the real story', *Humanist Magazine* (New York), 57 (2): pp. 7–9.

Ashcroft, R., Fraser, B., Kerr, M. and Ahmed, Z. (2001) 'Are antipsychotic drugs the right treatment for challenging behaviour in learning disability? The place of a randomised trial', *Journal of Medical Ethics* 27: 338–43.

Audit Commission (2002) *Forget Me Not: Mental Health Services for Older People.* London: Audit Commission.

Aware (1998) *Suicide in Ireland: A Global Perspective and a National Strategy.* Dublin: Aware Publications.

Balazs, J. (1993) 'Health care for single homeless people', pp. 51–93 in Fisher, K. and Collins, J. (eds), *Homelessness, Health Care and Welfare Provision.* London: Routledge.

Ball, J. A. (1994) *Reactions to Motherhood: the Role of Post-natal Care*, 2nd edn. Hull: Books for Midwives.

Banyard V. L. and Graham-Bermann S. A. (1998) 'Surviving poverty: stress and coping in the lives of housed and homeless mothers', *American Journal of Orthopsychiatry* 68 (3): 479–89.

Barker, P., Keady, J., Croom, S., Stevenson, C., Adams, T. and Reynolds, B. (1998) 'The Concept of Serious Mental Illness: Modern Myths and Grim Realities', *Journal of Psychiatric and Mental Health Nursing*, 5 (4): 247–54.

Barnes, C. (2000) 'A working social model? Disability work and disability politics in the 21st century', *Critical Social Policy* 20 (4): 441–57.

Barnes, C., Oliver, M. and Barton, L. (eds) (2002) *Disability Studies Today.* Cambridge: Polity.

Barnes, M. and Bowl, R. (2001) *Taking Over The Asylum: Empowerment and Mental Health*, Basingstoke: Palgrave.

Barnett, E. (1997) 'Collaboration and interdependence: care as a two way street', pp. 1–6 in Marshall, M. (ed.), *The State of the Art in Dementia Care.* London: Centre for Policy on Ageing.

Barnett, E. (2000) *Including the Person with Dementia in Designing and Delivering Care.* London: Jessica Kingsley.

Barry, M. (2001) 'Promoting positive mental health: theoretical frameworks for practice', *International Journal of Mental Health Promotion* 3 (1): 25–34.

Barry, M. M., O'Doherty, E. and Doherty, A. (1999) 'Mental health promotion in a rural context: research and realities from a community-based initiative in Northern Ireland'. *International Journal of Mental Health Promotion* 1 (1): 9–14.

Barry, M., Friel, S., Dempsey, C., Avalos, G. and Clarke, P. (2002) *Promoting Mental Health and Social Well-being: Cross-Border Opportunities and Challenges.* Armagh: Centre for Cross Border Studies and Dublin/Belfast: Institute of Public Health in Ireland.

Barton R. (1959) *Institutional Neurosis.* Bristol: Wright.

Bassuk, E. L. (1984) 'The homelessness problem', *Scientific American* 251: 40–5.

Bassuk E. L., Melnick S. and Browne A. (1998) 'Responding to the needs of low-income and homeless women who are survivors of family violence', *Journal of American Medical Women's Association* 53 (2): 57–64.

Bassuk, E. L., Rubin, L. and Lauriat, A. (1986) 'Characteristics of sheltered homeless families', *American Journal of Public Health* 76: 1097–1101.

Batt, V., Nic Gabhainn, S. and Falvey F. (2003) *Perspectives on the Provision of Counselling for Women in Ireland.* Dublin. Women's Health Council.

Baum C., Kennedy, D. L., Knapp, D. E., Juergens J. P. and G. A. Faich (1988) 'Prescription drug use in 1984 and changes over time', *Medical Care* 26: 105–14.

Bebbington , P. (1996) 'The origins of sex-differences in depressive disorder: bridging the gap', *International Review of Psychiatry* 8: 295–332.

Bennett, P. (2003) *Abnormal and Clinical Psychology.* Buckingham: Open University Press.

Beresford, P. (2002) 'Thinking about "mental health": towards a social model', *Journal of Mental Health* 11 (6): 581–4.

Bergin M. (1998) 'A descriptive study of the work of community psychiatric nurses', unpublished MMedSci thesis, Dublin: UCD.

Bergin, D. and Hunter, N. (2003) 'Medical concern grows on effects of new insanity bill', *Irish Medical News*, 26 May.

Berry, P. (2003) 'Psychodynamic therapy and intellectual disabilities: dealing with challenging behaviour', *International Journal of Disability, Development and Education* 50 (1): 39–51.

Bhugra, D. (1996) 'Young homeless and homeless families', pp. 41–58 in D. Bhugra (ed.), *Homelessness and Mental Health: Studies in Social and Community Psychiatry*, Cambridge, Cambridge University Press.

Bird, H. (1996) 'Epidemiology of childhood disorders in a cross-cultural context', *Journal of Child Psychology and Psychiatry* 37 (1): 35–49.

Blaikie, A. (1999) Ageing: old visions, new times? *The Lancet* (35) Supplement 4: SIV3

Blazer, D., Hughes, D. C. and George, L. K. (1991) 'The association of age and depression among the elderly: an epidemiologic exploration', *Journal of Gerontology* 46: M 210–15.

Blytheway, B. (2001) *Ageism*. Buckingham: Open University Press.

Bourne, E. (1998) *Healing Fear: New Approaches to Overcoming Anxiety*. Oakland, CA, New Harbinger.

Boxhill, N. and Beatty, A. (1987) 'Mother/child interaction among homeless women and their children in a public night shelter in Altanto, Georgia', *Child NS Youth Services*, 14 (1): 49–64

Bracton, H. (1915 [orig. 1569]) *De Legibus et Consuetudinibus Angliae*. Oxford: Oxford University Press.

Bradley, F., Smith, M., Long, J. and O'Dowd, T. (2002) 'Reported frequency of domestic violence: cross-sectional survey of women attending general practice', *British Medical Journal* 324: 271–4.

Breaky, W. (1996) 'Clinical work with homeless people in the USA', pp. 110–32 in Bhugra, D. (ed.), *Homelessness and Mental Health: Studies in Social and Community Psychiatry*, Cambridge: Cambridge University Press.

Breaky, W. R., Fischer, P. J., Kramer, M., Nestadt, G., Romanoski, A. J., Ross, A. et al. (1989) 'Health and mental health problems of homeless men and women in Baltimore', *Journal of the American Medical Association* 262: 1352–7.

Brenner, H. and Shelley, E. (1998) *Adding Years to Life and Life to Years: A Health Promotion Strategy for Older People*, Report no. 50. Dublin: National Council on Ageing and Older People and Health Promotion Unit.

Brodaty, H. (1988) 'Minimal brain damage in the adult II: Early dementia', *Patient Management* August: 127–50.

Brooke, S. (2002) 'Dedicated to dedicated provision', *Cornerstone* 11 (Dublin Homeless Agency): 14–19.

Brosnan, L., Collins, S., Dempsey, H., Dermody, F., Maguire, L. Maria, Morrin, N. (2002) *Pathways Report – Experiences of Mental Health Services from a User-led perspective*, Galway: Western Health Board and Schizophrenia Ireland.

Brown G. S. and Harris, T. (1978) *The Social Origins of Depression: A Study of Psychiatric Disorder in Women*. London: Tavistock/ NY: The Free Press.

Brown, P., Challis, D. and Von Abendorff, R. (1995) 'The work of a community mental health team for the elderly: referrals, caseloads, contact history and outcome', *International Journal of Geriatric Psychiatry* 11: 29–39.

Browne A. (1993) Family violence and homelessness: the relevance of trauma histories in the lives of homeless women', *American Journal of Orthopsychiatry* 63 (3): 370–84.

Browne, M. (1992) *Co-ordinating Services for the Elderly at Local Level: Swimming against the Tide. A Report on Two Pilot Projects.* Dublin: National Council for the Elderly.

Bryant, L. L., Corbett, K. K. and Kutner, J. S. (2001) 'In their own words: a model of healthy ageing', *Social Science and Medicine* 53: 927–41.

Brylewski, J. and Duggan, L. (1999) 'Antipsychotic medication for challenging behaviour in people with learning disability', *Journal of Intellectual Disability Research* 43: 360–71.

Burchardt, T., Le Grand, J. and Piachaud, D. (2002) 'Degrees of exclusion: developing a dynamic, multidimensional measure', pp. 30–43 in Hills, J., Le Grand, J. and Piachaud, D. (eds), *Understanding Social Exclusion.* Oxford: Oxford University Press.

Burke, H. (1987) *The People and the Poor Law in Nineteenth Century Ireland.* Littlehampton: WEB.

Burns, A., Dening, T. and Baldwin, R. (2001) 'Mental health problems', *British Medical Journal* 322: 789–91.

Busfield J. (1996) *Men, Women and Madness: Understanding Gender and Mental Disorder.* London: Macmillan.

Busfield J. (2001) 'Introduction: rethinking the sociology of mental health', pp. 1–16 in Busfield J. (ed.), *Rethinking the Sociology of Mental Health.* Oxford: Blackwell.

Byrne, R., Hogan, G. W. and McDermott, P. (1981) *Prisoners' Rights: A Study in Irish Prison Law.* Dublin: Co-op Books.

Cahill, S., Drury, M., Lawlor, B., O' Connor, D. and O' Connell, M. (2003) 'They have started to call it their club', *Dementia* 2 (1): 85–103.

Calkins, M. (1988) *Design for Dementia: Planning Environments for the Elderly and the Confused.* Owing Mills, MD: National Health Publishing.

Cameron, M., Edmans, Greatley, A. and Morris, D. (2003) *Community Renewal and Mental Health,* London: King's Fund.

Canetto, S. S. and Lester, D. (eds) (1995) *Women and Suicidal Behaviour.* New York: Springer.

Cantor, C. H. (2000) 'Suicide in the western world', pp. 9–28 in Hawton, K. and Van Heeringen, K. (eds), *The International Handbook of Suicide and Attempted Suicide.* Chichester: Wiley.

Cantor, C. H., Leenaars, A. A. and Lester, D. (1997) 'Under-reporting of Suicide in Ireland 1960–1989', *Archives of Suicide Research* 3: 5–12.

Carey, T. (2000) *Mountjoy: The Story of a Prison.* Cork: Collins.

Carey, T. (2004) 'Report of the Inspector of Mental Health Services 2003', in *Mental Health Commission's Annual Report 2003.* Dublin: Mental Health Commission.

Carr, A. (2000) 'Empirical studies of problems and treatment processes in children and adolescents', pp. 29–50 in Carr, A. (ed.), *Clinical Psychology in Ireland, Vol.* 3, pp 29–50.

Casey, P (2003) 'Most suicidal adolescents are ill', *The Irish Times,* 24 Sept.

Castel, R., Castel, F. and Lovell, A. (1982) *The Psychiatric Society,* New York: Columbia University Press.

Catholic Church (1994) *Catechism of the Catholic Church.* Veritas, Dublin.

Cattell, H. (2000) 'Suicide in the elderly'. *Advances in Psychiatric Treatment* 6: 102–8.

Challis, D. (2000) 'Case management and the care of people with dementia', pp. 46–56 in *Planning for Dementia Care in Ireland* (Conference Proceedings). National Council on Ageing and Older People.

Challis, D., Von Abendorff, R., Brown, P. and Chesterman, J. (1997) 'Care management and dementia: an evaluation of the Lewisham case management scheme', pp 139–64 in Hunter, S. (ed.), *Dementia: Challenges and New Directions.* London: Jessica Kingsley.

Champion L. A. and Power, M. J. (1995) 'Social and cognitive approaches to depression: towards a new synthesis', *British Journal of Clinical Psychology* 34: 485–503.

Cheston, R. and Bender, M. (1999) *Understanding Dementia: The Man with the Worried Eyes.* London: Jessica Kingsley.

Children's Rights Alliance (1998) *Children's Rights, Our Responsibilities.* Dublin: Children's Rights Alliance.

CHPS (2000) *General Healthcare Study of the Irish Prison Population.* Dublin: Stationery Office.

Clarke, B. (2004) 'Mental Health Commission and mental health services in Ireland', *Irish Social Worker* 22 (1): 17–18.

Clarke, J. (2001) 'Healthcare of refugees'. www. irishhealth. com.

Cleary, A. and Prizeman, G. (1998) *Homelessness and Mental Health.* Dublin: Social Science Research Centre.

Clinch, D. (1998) 'Do we need a new strategy for quality in health and welfare services for older people?', pp. 99–102 in *The Years Ahead: A Policy For the Elderly: Review of the Implementation of Recommendations of The Years Ahead – A Policy for the Elderly and Implications for Future Policy on Older People in Ireland,* report no 49. Dublin: National Council on Ageing and Older People.

Coakley, A. (2004a) 'Poverty and insecurity', pp. 112–27 in Fanning, B., Kennedy, P., Kiely, G. and Quin, S. (eds), *Theorising Irish Social Policy.* Dublin. UCD Press.

Coakley, A. (2004b) 'Mothers and poverty', in Kennedy, P. (ed.), *Motherhood in Ireland: Creation and Context.* Cork. Mercier.

Cohen, G., Binstock, R., Lynn, J., Lubitz. J., Neveloff-Dubler, N., Pelligrino, E., Perls, T., Scitovsky, A. and Weiner, J. (1997) *Seven Deadly Myths: Uncovering the Facts About the High Cost of the Last Year of Life.* Washington, DC: Alliance for Aging Research.

Cole, M. and Cole, S. R. (1996) *The Development of Children,* 3rd edn. New York: W. H. Freeman.

Collins, B. and McKeown, K. (1992) *Referral and Resettlement in the Simon Community,* Dublin: Simon Community National Office.

Commission on the Status of People with Disabilities (1996) *A Strategy for Equality.* Dublin: Stationery Office.

Committee of Inquiry into the Penal System (1985) *Report* (Whitaker Report). Dublin: Stationery Office.

Condon, D. (ed.) (2001) *Health and Dental Needs of Homeless People in Dublin.* Dublin: Northern Area Health Board.

Conlon C. (1999) *Women: The Picture of Health: A Review of Research on Women's Health in Ireland.* Dublin: Women's Health Council.

Conroy, P. and Fanagan, S. (2001) *Research Project on the Effective Recruitment of People with Disabilities into the Public Service, 2000.* Dublin: Equality Authority.

Convery J. (1998) 'Mental health social work with older people in the Republic of Ireland', pp. 171–89 in J. Campbell and R. Maveletelow (eds), *Mental Health Social Work, Comparative Issues in Policy and Practice.* Aldershot: Ashgate.

Council of Europe (1987) *European Prison Rules: Recommendation no. R (87)3 and Explanatory Memorandum.* Strasbourg: Council of Europe.

Council of Europe (1994) *European Rules on Community Sanctions and Measures: Recommendation no. R (92)16 and Explanatory Memorandum.* Strasbourg: Council of Europe.

Council of Europe (2000) http://www. coe. int/T/E/Legal_affairs/Legal_co-operation/Prisons_ and_alternatives/Legal_instruments/Rec. R (2000)22.

Council of Europe CPT (1999) *Report to the Irish Government on the visit to Ireland carried out by the European Committee for the Prevention of Torture and Inhuman or Degrading Treatment or Punishment (CPT) from 31 August to 9 September 1998.* Government of Ireland, Strasbourg/ Dublin.

Council of the European Union (1996) European Council of 29 Mar. 1996 concerning Community Action Programme on Health Promotion (1996–2000) (645/96/EC).

Council of the European Union (1999) Council Resolution of 18 Nov. 1999 on the Promotion of Mental Health (2000/C86/01).

Council of the European Union (2000) Article 152 of the Treaty on European Union (COM (2000/285 final).

Council of the European Union European Council (2000) of 16 May 2000 Communication on the Development of Public Health Policy, 16 May.

Courts Service (2004) *Annual Report.* Dublin: Courts Service.

Cowell, A. J., Broner, N. and Dupont, R. (2004) 'The cost-effectiveness of criminal justice diversion programs for people with serious mental illness co-occurring with substance abuse', *Journal of Contemporary Criminal Justice* 20 (3): 292–314.

Cox, G. and Lawless, M. (1999) *Wherever I Lay my Hat: A Study of Out of Home Drug Users.* Dublin: Merchant's Quay Project.

Crane, M. (1999) *Understanding Older Homeless People,* Buckingham: Open University Press.

Crisp, A. H., Gelder, M. G., Rix, S., Meltzer, H. I. and Rowlands, O. J. (2000) 'Stigmatisation of people with mental illnesses', *British Journal of Psychiatry* (177): 4–7.

Crowley, F. (2003) *Mental Illness: The Neglected Quarter.* Dublin: Amnesty International.

CSO (2002) *Quarterly National Household Survey – Disability in the Labour Force.* Second Quarter, Dublin.

CSO (2003) *Census of the Population 2002: Principal Demographic Results.* Dublin: Stationery Office.

CSO (2004a) *Population and Migration Estimates.* Dublin: Stationery Office.

CSO (2004b) *Quarterly National Household Survey: Disability Update,* quarter 1. Dublin: CSO.

Cumella, S., Grattan, E. and Vostanis, P. (1998) 'The mental health of children in homeless families and the contact with health education and social services', *Health and Social Care in the Community* 6 (5): 331–342.

Daatland, S. V. (1996) 'Caring for frail elderly people: policies in evolution', *Social Policy Studies* 19: 247–59.

Daly, A. and Walsh, D. (2001) *Activities of Irish Psychiatric Services 2000.* Dublin: HRB.

Daly, A.. and Walsh, D. (2002) *Irish Psychiatric Hospitals and Units Census, 2001.* Dublin: HRB.

Daly, A. and Walsh, D. (2003) *Activities of Irish Psychiatric Services 2001.* Dublin: HRB.

Daly, A., Walsh, D., Moran, R. and O' Doherty, Y. K. (2004) *Activities of Irish Psychiatric Services 2003.* Dublin: HRB.

Daly, M. (1993) *Abandoned: Profile of Europe's Homeless People.* Brussels: European Federation of National Organisations working with the Homeless.

De Groef, J. and Heinemann E. (1999) *Psychoanalysis and Mental Handicap,* London: Free Association Books.

Delaney, S., Garavan, R. and Mc Gee, H. (2001) *Care and Case Management for Older People in Ireland*, Report no. 66. Dublin: National Council on Ageing and Older People.

DeLeo, D., Bertolote, J. and Lester, D. (2002) 'Self-directed violence', in Krug, E.G. et al. (eds), *World Report on Violence and Health*. Geneva: WHO.

Denihan, A., Kirby, M., Bruce, I., Cunningham, C., Coakley, D. and Lawlor, B. A. (2000) 'Three-year prognosis of depression in the community-dwelling elderly', *British Journal of Psychiatry* 176: 453–7.

Department for International Development (2000) *Disability, Poverty and Development*. London: DFID.

Department of Education (2001) *Educational Provision and Support for Persons with Autism Spectrum Disorders: The Report of the Task Force on Autism*. Dublin: Stationery Office.

Department of Environment and Local Government (2000) *Homelessness: An Integrated Strategy*. Dublin: Stationery Office.

Department of Environment and Local Government (2002) *Homeless Preventative Strategy*. Dublin: Stationery Office.

Department of Health (1945) *Mental Health Act*. Dublin: Stationery Office.

Department of Health (1966) *Commission of Inquiry into Mental Illness*. Dublin: Stationery Office.

Department of Health (1984) *The Psychiatric Services: Planning for the Future*. Dublin: Stationery Office.

Department of Health (1988) *The Years Ahead: A Policy for the Elderly*. Dublin: Stationery Office.

Department of Health (1990) *Health (Nursing Home) Act*. Dublin: Stationery Office.

Department of Health (1992) *Green Paper on Mental Health*. Dublin: Stationery Office.

Department of Health (1994a) *Services for Persons with Autism*. Dublin: Stationery Office.

Department of Health (1994b) *Shaping a Healthier Future: A Strategy for Effective Healthcare in the 1990s*. Dublin: Stationery Office.

Department of Health (1995a) *A Health Promotion Strategy*. Dublin: Stationery Office.

Department of Health (1995b) *A New Mental Health Act, White Paper*. Dublin: Stationery Office.

Department of Health (1996) *Discussion Document on the Mental Health Needs of Persons with Mental Handicap (Mulcahy Report)*. Dublin: Stationery Office.

Department of Health and Children (1990) The Health (Nursing Homes) Act. Dublin: Stationery Office.

Department of Health and Children (1998a) *Guidelines on Good Practice and Quality Assurance in Mental Health Services*. Dublin: Stationery Office.

Department of Health and Children (1998b) *Report of the National Task Force on Suicide*. Dublin: Stationery Office.

Department of Health and Children (1999) *Best Health for Children: Developing a Partnership with Families* Dublin: Stationery Office.

Department of Health and Children (2000a) *National Children's Strategy: Our Children, Their Lives*. Dublin: Stationery Office.

Department of Health and Children (2000b) *National Health Promotion Strategy 2000–2005*. Dublin: Stationery Office.

Department of Health and Children (2001a) *First Report of the Working Group on Child and Adolescent Psychiatric Services*. Dublin: Stationery Office.

Department of Health and Children (2001b) *Quality and Fairness: A Health System for You*. Dublin: Stationery Office.

Department of Health and Children (2001c) *Our Children: Their Lives.* Dublin: Stationery Office.

Department of Health and Children (2001d) *Mental Health Act.* Dublin: Stationery Office.

Department of Health and Children (2001e) *Primary Care: A New Direction.* Dublin: Stationery Office.

Department of Health and Children (2001f) *Your Views about Health, Report on Consultation, Quality and Fairness: A Health System for You, Health Strategy.* Dublin: Stationery Office.

Department of Health and Children (2001g) *Youth Homelessness Strategy.* Dublin: Stationery Office.

Department of Health and Children (2002) *Action Plan for People Management in the Health Service.* Dublin: Stationery Office.

Department of Health and Children (2003a) *Health Statistics, 2002.* Dublin: Stationery Office.

Department of Health and Children (2003b) *Quality and Fairness: A Health System for You: Action Plan Progress Report.* Dublin: Stationery Office.

Department of Health and Children (2003c) *Working Group on Child and Adolescent Psychiatric Services: Second Report.* Dublin: Stationery Office.

Department of Health and Children (2003d) *Report of the Inspector of Mental Hospitals for the year ending 31st December, 2002.* Dublin: Stationery Office.

Department of Health and Children (2004a) *Outline Sectoral Plan under the Disability Bill 2004.* Dublin: Stationery Office.

Department of Health and Children (2004b) *Report of the Inspector of Mental Hospitals for the Year Ending 31st December 2003.* Dublin: Stationery Office.

Department of Health and Children (2004c) *Review of the National Health Promotion Strategy 2004.* Dublin: Stationery Office.

Department of Health, Social Services and Public Safety, Northern Ireland (2003) *Promoting Mental Health Strategy and Action Plan 2003–2008.* Belfast: Department of Health, Social Services and Public Safety Northern Ireland.

Department of Justice (1947) *Rules for the Government of Prisons* (Statutory Rules and Orders, 1947 no. 320). Dublin: Stationery Office.

Department of Justice (1983) *Annual Report on the Prisons and Places of Detention.* Dublin: Stationery Office.

Department of Justice (1990) *Annual Report on the Prisons and Places of Detention.* Dublin: Stationery Office.

Department of Justice (1994) *The Management of Offenders: A Five Year Plan.* Dublin: Stationery Office.

Department of Justice (1997) *Tackling Crime: Discussion Paper.* Dublin: Stationery Office.

Department of Justice, Equality and Law Reform (1999a) *Report of the National Steering Group on Deaths in Prisons.* Dublin: Stationery Office.

Department of Justice, Equality and Law Reform (1999b) *National Disability Authority Act.* Dublin: Stationery Office.

Department of Justice, Equality and Law Reform (1999c) *Towards Equal Citizenship: Progress Report on the Implementation of the Recommendations of the Commission on the Status of People with Disabilities,* Dublin: Stationery Office.

Department of Justice Equality and Law Reform (2000) *Review of the Coroner Service.* Dublin: Stationery Office.

Department of Justice, Equality and Law Reform (2001) *Disability Bill.* Dublin: Stationery Office.

Department of Justice, Equality and Law Reform (2003) *Community Security and Equality. Strategy Statement 2003–2005.* Dublin: Stationery Office.

Department of Social and Family Affairs (2000) *Comhairle Act.* Dublin: Stationery Office.

Department of the Taoiseach (2003) *Sustaining Progress Social Partnership Agreement 2003–2005.* Dublin: Stationery Office.

Departments of State and Official Bodies and Royal Commission on the Law Relating to Mental Illness and Mental Deficiency (1957) *Royal Commission on the Law Relating to Mental Illness and Mental Deficiency, 1954–1957: Report.* London: HMSO.

Desjarlais, R., Eisenberg, L., Good, B. and Kleinman, A. (1996) *World Mental Health: Problems and Priorities in Low-Income Countries.* Oxford: Oxford University Press.

Deveraux, D. (2000) 'A psychological service for refugees and asylum seekers: some theoretical and practical considerations'. *Éisteach* 2 (14): 9–13.

Diekstra, R. W. F. (1993) 'The epidemiology of suicide and para suicide', *Acta Psychiatrica Scandanavica,* Suppl. 371: 9–20.

Diffley, C. (2003) *Managing Mental Health.* London: The Work Foundation and Mind.

Digby, P. W. (1976) *Hostels and Lodgings for Single People.* London: HMSO.

Ditton, P. M. (1999) *Mental Health and Treatment of Inmates and Probationers: Special Report.* Washington DC: Department of Justice, Bureau of Justice Statistics.

Dogra, N., Parkin, A., Gale, F. and Frake, C. (2002) *A Multidisciplinary Handbook of Child and Adolescent Mental Health for Front-line Professionals.* London: Jessica Kingsley.

Doherty, K., Fitzgerald, M. and Matthews, P. (2003) 'Services for autism in Ireland' in Fitzgerald, M. (ed.), *Irish Families Under* Stress, vol. 7. Dublin: South Western Area Health Board.

Donnelly, M. (1992) *The Politics of Mental Health in Italy.* London: Routledge.

Dooley, C. (2003) 'Job scheme expansion likely to be restricted', *The Irish Times,* 30 Sept. 2003.

Dooley, E. (1995) *Homicide in Ireland 1972–1991.* Dublin: Stationery Office.

Downer, R. (2001) *Homelessness and its Consequences: The Impact on Children's Psychological Well-being.* New York: Routledge.

Downs, M. (2000) 'The role of the general practitioner in dementia care' in *Planning for Dementia Care in Ireland, Conference Proceedings,* Report no. 56. Dublin: National Council on Ageing and Older People.

Doyal, L (1995) *What Makes Women Sick? Gender and the Political Economy of Health.* New Brunswick, NJ: Rutgers University Press.

Doyal L. and Gough, I. (1991) *A Theory of Human Need.* London: Macmillan.

Drake, R. E., Osher F. C. and Wallach M. A. (1991) 'Homelessness and dual diagnosis', *American Psychologist* 46 (11): 1149–58.

Drake, R. E., Wallach, M. A. and Hoffman, J. S. (1989) 'Housing instability and homelessness among aftercare patients of an urban state hospital', *Hospital and Community Psychiatry* 40: 46–51.

Dual Diagnosis Recovery Network (1996) Available www.dualdiagnosis.org

Dublin Simon Community (2003a) 'It's hard to understand why people who are homeless are still denied the chance of a decent home', *Annual Report 2002/3.* Dublin: Dublin Simon Community.

Dublin Simon Community (2003b) *Dublin Simon Community Annual Report 2002/2003*. Dublin: Simon Community.

Eastern Regional Health Authority (2002a) *Strategic Action Plan on Youth Homelessness*. Dublin: Eastern Regional Health Authority.

Eastern Regional Health Authority (2002b) *Review of Persons with Autistic Spectrum Disorders*. Dublin: Eastern Regional Health Authority.

Eccles, M., Clarke, J., Livingston, M., Freemantle, N. and Mason, J. (1998) 'North of England evidence-based guidelines development project: guidelines for the primary care management of dementia', *British Medical Journal* 317: 802–8.

Edgar, B. and Doherty, J. (2001) 'Introduction', in Edgar, B. and Doherty, J. (eds), *Women and Homelessness in Europe: Pathways, Services and Experiences*. Bristol: Policy Press.

Edwards S. D. (2001) *Philosophy of Nursing: An Introduction*. Basingstoke: Palgrave.

Elliott, I. (2001) *Health Impact Assessment: An Introductory Paper*. Dublin and Belfast: Institute of Public Health in Ireland.

Enkin M., Keirse, M., Renfrew, M. and Neilson J. (1995) *A Guide to Effective Care in Pregnancy and Childbirth*, 2nd edn. Oxford: Oxford University Press.

Equality Authority (2002) *Implementing Equality for Older People*. Dublin: Stationery Office.

Esping-Andersen, G. (1990) *The Three Worlds of Welfare Capitalism*. Cambridge: Polity.

Esping-Andersen, G. (1996) *Welfare States in Transition*. London: Sage.

European Commission (2001) 'Attitudes of Europeans to disability', *Eurobarometer* 54 (2).

European Commission (2002) *Employment in Europe 2002 Recent Trends and Prospects*. Luxembourg: European Commission.

European Commission (2003) *The Social Situation in the European Union*. Luxembourg: European Commission.

European Network on Mental Health Policy (1997) *Framework for Action for Promoting Mental Health in Europe*. Brussels: European Commission.

European Union (2000) Council Directive 2000/78/EC of 27 Nov., L303, 2. 12. 2000, Luxembourg: OOPEC.

European Women's Lobby (1999) *Presenting Women's Perspectives on Key Issues to the European Union*. Brussels: Author.

Fahey, T. and Murray, P. (1994) *Health and Autonomy Among the Over-65s in Ireland*. Report no. 39. Dublin: National Council for the Elderly.

Fakhoury W. and Priebe S. (2002) 'The process of deinstitutionalization: an international overview', *Current Opinion in Psychiatry* (15): 187–92.

Fanning, B. (2002) *Racism and Social Change in the Republic of Ireland*. Manchester: Manchester University Press.

Fanning, B. (2004a) 'Asylum-seeker and migrant children in Ireland: racism, institutional neglect and social work', pp. 201–16 in Hayes, D. and Humphries, B. (eds), *Social Work, Immigration and Asylum: Debates, Dilemmas and Ethical Issues for Social Work and Social Care Practice*. London: Jessica Kingsley.

Fanning, B. (2004b) 'Locating Irish social policy', pp. 6–22 in Fanning, B., Kennedy, P., Kiely G. and Quin, S. (eds), *Theorising Irish Social Policy*. Dublin: UCD Press.

FÁS (2003) *FÁS Quarterly Labour Market Commentary*, Summer. Dublin: FÁS.

Faulkner, A. (2000) *Strategies for Living: A Report of User-Led Research into People's Strategies for Living with Mental Disorder*. London: Mental Health Foundation.

Feeney, A., McGee, H., Holohan, T. and Shannon, W. (2000) *Health of Hostel-Dwelling Men in Dublin*. Dublin: Royal College of Surgeons in Ireland and Eastern Health Board.

Fennell, G. C., Phillipson, C. and Evers H. (1988) *The Sociology of Old Age*. Milton Keynes: Open University Press.

Ferguson, D., Horwood, J. L and Beautrais A. L. (1999) 'Is sexual orientation related to mental health problems and suicidality in young people?' *Archives of General Psychiatry* 56: 876–80.

Fernandez, J. (1996) 'Homelessness: an Irish perspective', pp 209–29 in Bhugra, D. (ed.), *Homelessness and Mental Health*. Cambridge: Cambridge University Press.

Fernandez, J. (2003) 'Caring for the homeless mentally ill: status and directions', Seminar presented for the Irish Psychiatric Association, St Patrick's Hospital, Dublin.

Fernando, S. (2002) *Mental Health, Race and Culture*, 2nd edn. Basingstoke: Palgrave.

Finlay, R. and Reynolds, J. (1987) *Social Work and Refugees: A Handbook on Working with People in Exile in the UK*. Cambridge: National Extension College/Refugee Action.

Fitzgerald, E. (2000) 'Community services for independence in old age: rhetoric and reality. follow the money trail', *Administration* 48 (3): 75–89.

Fitzgerald, M. (1991) *Irish Families Under Stress*, vol. 4. Dublin: Eastern Health Board.

Fitzgerald, M. and Corvin, A. (2003) 'Diagnosis and differential diagnosis of Asperger's Syndrome' in Fitzgerald, M (ed.), *Irish Families Under Stress*, vol. 7. Dublin: South Western Area Health Board.

Focus Ireland (2003) *Health and Homelessness: A Series of 10 Modules for the Nursing Degree Programme*. Dublin: Focus Ireland.

Focus Ireland, the Mater Hospital and the Northern Area Health Board (2000) *The Mental and Physical Health and Well-Being of Homeless Families in Ireland: A Pilot Study*. Dublin: Focus Ireland.

Fombonne, E. (1995) 'Eating disorders: time trends and possible explanatory mechanisms', pp. 616–83 Rutter, M. and Smith, D. J. (eds), *Psychosocial Disorders in Young People: Time Trends and Their Causes*. Chichester: Wiley.

Forum for People with Disabilities (2001) *Advocacy: A Rights Issue*. Dublin: Forum for People with Disabilities.

Foucault, M. (1961) *Madness and Civilization: A History of Insanity in the Age of Reason*. London: Routledge.

Friedli, L. (2003) *Making it Effective: A Guide to Evidence-Based Mental Health Promotion*. London: Mentality UK.

Friel, S., Nic Gabhainn, S. and Kelleher, C. (1999) *The National Lifestyle Surveys: Survey of Lifestyle, attitudes and Nutrition (Slán) and The Irish Health Behaviour in School-Aged Children Survey*. Dublin: Department of Health and Children.

Fryers, T., Melzer, D. and Jenkins, R. (2003) 'Social inequalities and the common mental disorders: a systematic review of the evidence', *Social Psychiatry and Psychiatric Epidemiology* 38 (5): 229–37.

Galen, C. G. (1997) 'Mixtures' Book II, in *Selected Works*, trans. Singer, P. N. Oxford: Oxford University Press.

Gallant S. J and P. S Derry (1995) 'Menarche, menstruation and menopause, psychosocial research and future directions', pp. 199–259 in Stanton, L. A. and Gallant, S. J. (eds), *Psychology and Women's Health Progress and Challenges in Research and Application*. Washington DC: American Psychological Association.

Garavan, R., Winder, R. and Mc Gee, H. (2001) *Health and Social Services for Older People (HeSSOP). Consulting Older People on Health and Social Services: A Survey of Service Use, Experiences and Needs*, Report no. 64. Dublin: National Council on Ageing and Older People.

Garrison, P. (2004) 'Children, mental health and human rights: an international perspective', *Representing Children* 16 (4): 224–36.

Gavigan P. and McKeon, P. (1995) *Public Attitudes to the Treatment of Depression in General Practices*. Dublin: Abstracts of World Congress of World Federation of Mental Health.

Gillberg, C. (1991) 'Clinical and neurobiological aspects of Asperger's syndrome in six families studied', pp. 122–46 in Frith, U. (ed.), *Autism and Asperger's Syndrome*. Cambridge: Cambridge University Press.

Gilligan, C (1982) *In a Different Voice*, Cambridge, MA: Harvard University Press.

Goffman, E. (1961) *Asylums*. New York: Doubleday.

Gogarty, M. (1998) *Disability Equality: Guidelines for Union Negotiators*. Dublin: Irish Trade Union Trust.

Goldberg, D. and Huxley, P. (1980) *Mental Illness in the Community: The Pathway to Psychiatric Care*. London: Tavistock.

Goldberg, D. and Huxley, P. (1992) *Common Mental Disorders: A Bio-Social Model*. London: Routledge.

Goldsmith. M. (1996) *Hearing the Voice of People with Dementia: Opportunities and Obstacles*. London: Jessica Kingsley.

Goodley, D. (2000) *Self Advocacy in the Lives of People with Learning Disabilities*. Buckingham: Open University Press.

Goodwin S. (1997) *Comparative Mental Health Policy: From Institutional to Community Care*. London: Sage.

Government of Ireland (1945) *Mental Treatment Act*. Dublin: Stationery Office.

Government of Ireland (1991) *Child Care Act*. Dublin: Stationery Office.

Government of Ireland (1996) *Health (Amendment) (no. 3) Act 1996*. Dublin: Stationery Office.

Government of Ireland (1997) *Sharing in Progress: National Anti-Poverty Strategy* Dublin: Stationery Office.

Government of Ireland (1998) *The Good Friday Agreement*. Dublin: Stationery Office.

Government of Ireland (2001) *Mental Health Act*. Dublin: Stationery Office.

Gunnell, D., Middleton, N., Whitley, E. Dorling, D and Frankel, S. (2003) 'Influence of cohort effects on patterns of suicide in England and Wales, 1950–1999', *British Journal of Psychiatry* 182: 164–70.

Guy, W. A. (1869) 'On insanity and crime; and on the plea of insanity in criminal cases', *Journal of the Statistical Society* 32: 159–91.

Halpenny A. M., Greene S., Hogan D., Smith M. and McGee H. (2001) *Children of Homeless Mothers. The Daily Life Experiences and Wellbeing of Children in Homeless Families*. Dublin: Royal College of Surgeons in Ireland and Children's Research Centre, TCD.

Handy, J. A. (1982) 'Psychological and social aspects of induced abortion', *Clinical Psychologist Journal* 1: 29.

Hanly, C. (1999) *An Introduction to Irish Criminal Law*. Dublin: Gill & Macmillan.

Hannigan B. and Cutcliffe J. (2002) 'Challenging contemporary mental health policy: time to assuage the coercion?', *Journal of Advanced Nursing* 37 (5): 477–84.

Hargreaves, D. and Tiggermann, M. (2003) 'The effect of "thin ideal" television commercials on body dissatisfaction and schema activation during early adolescence', *Journal of Youth and Adolescence* 32 (5): 367–73.

Harper, G. and Chitty, C. (2004) *The Impact of Corrections on Re-offending: A Review of 'What Works'*, Home Office Research Study 291. London: Home Office.

Hartwell, S. (2004) 'Triple stigma: persons with mental illness and substance abuse problems in the criminal justice system', *Criminal Justice Policy Review* 15 (1): 84–99.

Harvey, B. (1998) *Homelessness and Mental Health, Policies and Services in an Irish and European Context*. Dublin: Homelessness and Mental Health Action Group.

Haslam, C., Brown, S., Hastings, S. and Haslam, R. (2003) *Effects of Prescribed Medication on Performance in the Working Population*, Research Report 05. London: Health and Safety Executive.

Hautala, H. (1999) *Report on Women's Health Status: Second Report to the Committee on Women's Rights*. Luxembourg: European Commission.

Hawton, K. and Van Heeringen, K. (eds), *The International Handbook of Suicide and Attempted Suicide*. Chichester/New York: Wiley.

Health Education Authority, UK (1997) *Mental Health Promotion: A Quality Framework*. London: HEA.

Health Education Board for Scotland (2001) *Mental Health Promotion: Strategic Statement*. Edinburgh: Health Education Board for Scotland.

Health Promotion Agency Northern Ireland (1999) *Mental Health Promotion: A Database of Initiatives in Northern Ireland*. Belfast: Health Promotion Agency Northern Ireland.

Hearn, J. (1998) *The Violences of Men*. London: Sage.

Heath, I (2001) 'Domestic violence as a women's health issue', *Women's Health Issues* 11 (4): 376–81.

Heller, T. and Heller, L. (2003) 'First among equals: does drug treatment for dementia claim more than its fair share of resources'. *Dementia* 2 (1): 7–19.

Hensey B. (1988) *The Health Services of Ireland*, 4th edn. Dublin: IPA.

Herrell, R., Goldberg, J., True, R., Ramakrishnan, V., Lyons, M., Eisen, S. and Tsuang, T. (1999) 'Sexual orientation and suicidality: a co-twin study in adult men', *Archives of General Psychiatry* 56: 867–74.

Herron S. (1997) 'The cloudy waters of mental health', pp. 171–7 in Trent D. R. and Reed C. A. (eds), *Promotion of Mental Health*, vol. 6. Aldershot: Ashgate.

Herron, S. and Mortimer, R. (1999) 'Mental health': a contested concept', *International Journal of Mental Health Promotion* 1 (1): 4–8.

Hickey T., Moran R. and Walsh D. (2003) *Psychiatric Day Care: An Underused Option? The Purposes and Functions of Psychiatric Day Hospitals and Day Centres: A Study in Two Health Boards*. Dublin: HRB.

Higgs, P., Hyde, M., Wiggins, R. and Blane, B. (2003) 'Researching quality of life in early old age: the importance of the sociological dimension' *Social Policy and Administration* 37 (3): 239–52.

Hill, A., O'Donnchadha, G. and O'Connor D. (2003) *A Survey of Perceived Stress Levels and Coping Responses in 1st Year Post-Primary School Students*. Kerry: Kerry Mental Health Association.

Hills, J., Le Grand, J. and Piachaud, D. (eds) (2002) *Understanding Social Exclusion*. Oxford: Oxford University Press.

Hodgson, R. J. and Abbasi, T (1995) *Effective Mental Health Promotion: Literature Review.* Technical Report no. 13 Cardiff: Health Promotion Wales.

Hoffman, E. and Massion, C. (2000) 'Women's health as a medical speciality and a clinical science', pp. 3–16 in Sherr, L. and St Lawrence, J. (eds), *Women, Health and the Mind.* Chichester: Wiley.

Holburn, S. and Vietze, P. E. (2002) *Person Centred Planning: Research, Practice and Future Directions.* Baltimore: Paul H. Brookes.

Holohan, T. (1997) *Health Service Utilisation and Barriers to Health Service Utilisation Among the Adult Homeless Population of Dublin.* Dublin: Eastern Health Board.

Homeless Agency (2004) *Making it Home: An Action Plan on Homelessness in Dublin 2004–2006.* Dublin: Homeless Agency.

Homeless Preventative Strategy (2002) Dublin: Government of Ireland.

Honn Qualls, S. (2002) 'Defining mental health in later life', *Generations* Spring: 9–13.

Hopper, K. (1989) 'Deviance and dwelling space: notes on the resettlement of homeless persons with alcohol and drug problems', *Contemporary Drug Problems* 16: 391–414.

Horton, R. (1997) 'Ageing today and tomorrow', *The Lancet* 350 (9085) 1156–7.

Hosman, C and Jane-Llopis, E. (2000) Chapter 3 in *The Evidence of Health Promotion Effectiveness, Shaping Public Health in a New Europe. Part Two Evidence Book*, 2nd edn. Brussels-Luxembourg: European Commission.

Hosman, C. M. H. (2000) 'Prevention and health promotion on the international scene: The need for a more effective and comprehensive approach', *Addictive Behaviours* 25 (6): 943–54.

Houghton, F. T. and Hickey, C. (2000) *Focusing on B&Bs: The Unacceptable Growth of Emergency B&B Placement in Dublin.* Dublin: Focus Ireland.

HRB (1997) *Annual Report of the National Intellectual Disability Database Committee, 1996.* Dublin: HRB.

HRB (2003) *Annual Report of the National Intellectual Disability Database Committee, 2001.* Dublin: HRB.

HRB (2004) *Activities of the Irish Psychiatric Services, 2003.* Dublin, HRB.

Hugman, R. (1994) *Ageing and the Care of Older People in Europe.* New York: St Martin's.

Huxley, P. (1997) 'Mental health', pp. 133–8 in Davies, M. (ed.), *The Blackwell Companion To Social Work.* Oxford: Blackwell.

Iacono, T. and Murray, V. (2003) 'Issues of informed consent in conducting medical research involving people with intellectual disability', *Journal of Applied Research in Intellectual Disabilities* 16: 41–51.

Iliffe, S. (1994) 'Why GPs have a bad reputation', *Journal of Dementia Care* Nov./Dec.24–5.

Illovsky, M. E. (2003) *Mental Health Professionals, Minorities and the Poor.* New York: Brunner-Routledge.

ILO (2000) *Mental Health in the Workplace: Executive Summary.* Geneva: ILO.

ILO (2001) *Mental Health in the Workplace, Situation analysis – United States.* Geneva: ILO.

Immigrant Council of Ireland (2003) *Labour Migration into Ireland.* Dublin: Immigrant Council of Ireland.

Ineichen, B. (1990) 'The extent of dementia among old people in residential care', *International Journal of Geriatric Psychiatry* 5: 327–35.

Inspector of Mental Health Services (2004) *First Report.* Dublin: Stationery Office.

Inspector of Mental Hospitals (2003) *Report for the year ending 31st December 2002.* Dublin: Stationery Office.

Inspector of Prisons and Places of Detention (2004) *First Annual Report for the Years 2002–2003.* Dublin Department of Justice, Equality and Law Reform.

Interdepartmental Committee (1968) *The Care of the Aged.* Dublin: Stationery Office.

Interdepartmental Committee on Mentally Ill and Maladjusted Persons (1978) *Treatment and Care of Persons Suffering from Mental Disorder Who Appear before the Courts on Criminal Charges.* Dublin: Stationery Office.

IPS (2001) *Annual Report.* Dublin: Irish Prison Service.

IPS (2003) *Annual Report.* Dublin: Irish Prison Service.

Irish Advocacy Network (2003) Irish Advocacy Network 2003 (online) Available: www. irishadvocacynetwork. com.

Irish Association of Suicidology (2004) *Suicide and Older People: Proceedings of the Eighth Annual Conference.* Irish Association of Suicidology.

Irish College of Psychiatrists (2002) *Position Statement on Psychiatric Services for Adolescents,* Dublin: ICP.

Irish College of Psychiatrists (2003a) http://mentalhealthpolicy. ie/submissions/submission102. pdf.

Irish College of Psychiatrists (2003b) *Psychotherapy Services: A strategy for Ireland.* Dublin: ICP.

Irish College of Psychiatrists (2003c) *Submission to the Expert Group on Mental Health Services.* Dublin: ICP.

Irish College of Psychiatrists (2004a) *Presentation to the Joint Committee on Health and Children.* Dublin: ICP.

Irish College of Psychiatrists (2004b) *Submission to the Expert Group on Mental Health Policy.* Dublin: ICP.

Irish Psychiatric Association (2003) *'The Stark Facts': The Need for a Mental Health Strategy as well as Resources.* Dublin: Irish Psychiatric Association.

The Irish Times (2004) 'Unstable man held after series of London knife attacks', 24 Dec.

Jacob, B. and Greene, J. (1998) *In-Patient Child Psychiatry: Modern Practice, Research and the Future.* London: Routledge.

Jamieson, L. and Taylor, P. J. (2004) 'A re-conviction study of special (high security) hospital patients', *British Journal of Criminology* 44: 783–802.

Jané-Llopes, E. (2004) 'Prevention and promotion in mental health for children and adolescents: a policy approach', paper presented at WHO Pre-Conference on Mental Health of Children and Adolescents.

Jenkins, R. Lehtinen, V. and Lahtinen, E. (2000) 'Emerging perspectives on mental health', *International Journal of Mental Health Promotion* 3 (1): 8–12.

Jones K., Brown J. and Bradshaw J. (1978) *Issues in Social Policy.* London: Routledge & Kegan Paul.

Jones, J. M., Bennett, S., Olmsted, M. P., Lawson, M. L. and Rodin, G. (2001) 'Disordered eating attitudes and behaviours in teenaged girls: a school-based study', *Canadian Medical Association Journal* 165 (5): 547–52.

Jorm, A. F., Korten, A. E. and Henderson, A. S. (1987) 'The prevalence of dementia: a quantitative integration of the literature', *Acta Psychiatrica Scandinavica* 76: 465–79.

Judd, S., Marshall, M. and Phippen, P. (1998) 'Design for dementia', *Journal of Dementia Care,* pp. 11–14.

Kalache, A. and Kickbusch, I. (1997) 'A global strategy for healthy ageing' *World Health* 4: 4–5.

Kansi, J., Wichstrøm, L. and Bergman, L. R. (2003) 'Eating problems and the self-concept: results based on a representative sample of Norwegian adolescent girls', *Journal of Youth and Adolescence* 32 (5): 325–35.

Katona, C. and Robertson, M. (2000) *Psychiatry at a Glance,* Oxford: Blackwell.

Katschnig, H. (1997) 'How useful is the concept of quality of life in psychiatry?' pp. 3–15 in Katschnig, H., Freeman, H. and Sartorius, M. (eds), *Quality of Life in Mental Disorders.* New York: Wiley.

Kellegher, P., Kellegher, C. and Corbett, M. (2000) *Left Out on Their Own: Young People Leaving Care in Ireland,* Dublin: Oak Tree.

Kelleher, M. J (1991) 'Suicide in Ireland', *Irish Medical Journal* 84 (2): 40–4.

Kelleher, M. J. (1996) *Suicide and the Irish.* Cork: Mercier.

Kelleher, M. J., Corcoran, P. and Keeley, H. S. (1997) 'Suicide in Ireland: statistical, social and clinical considerations', *Archives of Suicide Research* 3: 13–24.

Kelley, A. E., Schochet, T. and Landry, C. F. (2004) 'Adolescent brain development: vulnerabilities and opportunities', *Annals of the New York Academy of Sciences* 1021: pp. 27–32.

Kelly, F. (1988) *A Guide to Early Irish Law.* Dublin: Institute for Advanced Studies.

Kennedy, G. J., Kelman, H. R., Thomas, C., Wisniewski, W., Metz, H. and Bijur, P. E. (1989) 'Hierarchy of characteristics associated with depressive symptoms in an urban elderly sample', *American Journal of Psychiatry* 146: 220–5.

Kennedy P. (2002) *Maternity in Ireland: A Woman Centred Perspective.* Dublin: Liffey.

Kennedy, P. (ed.) (2004) *Motherhood in Ireland: Creation and Context.* Cork: Mercier.

Kennedy, S. (1985) *But Where Can I Go? Homeless Women in Dublin.* Dublin: Arlen House.

Keogh F., Finnerty A., O'Grady Walshe A., Daly I., Murphy D., Lane A. and Walsh D. (2003) 'Meeting the needs of people with schizophrenia living in the community: a report from a European collaboration', *Irish Journal of Psychological Medicine* 20 (2): 45–51.

Keogh, F. and Roche, A. (1996) *Mental Disorders in Older Irish People: Incidence, Prevalence and Treatment,* Report no. 45. Dublin: National Council for the Elderly.

Kerkhof, A. (2003) Paper presented to Irish Association of Suicidology Conference, Killarney, 21 Nov.

Killick, J. and Allan, K. (2001) *Communication and the Care of People with Dementia.* Buckingham: Open University Press.

Kirby, M. (2003) 'Is late onset depression a harbinger of dementia?', *Irish Psychiatrist* 4 (3): 88–9.

Kitwood, T. (1997) *Dementia Reconsidered: The Person Comes First.* Buckingham: Open University Press.

Klaczynski, P. A., Goold, K. W. and Mudry, J. J. (2004) 'Culture obesity stereotypes, self-esteem and the 'thin ideal': a social identity perspective', *Journal of Youth and Adolescence* 33 (4): 307–17.

Koegel, P. and Burnam, M. A. (1988) 'Alcoholism among homeless adults in the inner city of Los Angeles', *Archives of General Psychiatry* 45: 1011–18.

Kohen, M (2003) 'Gender sensitive psychiatric services', Presentation at Consultative Event held at Wigan Investment Centre, UK.

Koss, M. P., Goodman, L. A., Browne, A., Fitzgerald, L. F., Keita G. P. and Russo, N. F. (1994) *No Safe Haven: Male Violence Against Women at Home, at Work and in the Community,*.Washington DC: American Psychological Association.

Lahtinen, E., Lehtinen, V., Riikonen, E. and Ahonen, J. (eds) (1999) *Framework for Promoting Mental Health in Europe*. Helsinki: National Research and Development Centre for Welfare and Health (STAKES).

Lam, D. H., Chan, N. and Leff, J. (1995) 'Family work for schizophrenia: some issues for Chinese immigrant families', *Journal of Family Therapy* 17: 281–97.

Lamb, H. and Lamb, D. (1990) 'Factors contributing to homelessness among the chronically and severely mentally ill', *Hospital and Community Psychiatry* 41: 301–4.

Lang C., Field T., Pickens J., Martinez A., Bendell D., Yando R. and Routh D. (1996) 'Preschoolers of dysphoric mothers', *Journal Child Psychology and Psychiatry* 37 (2): 221–4.

Lavikainen, J., Lahtinen, E. and Lehtinen, V. (eds) (2001) *Public Health Approach on Mental Health in Europe*. Helsinki: National Research and Development Centre for Welfare and Health (STAKES).

Lawlor, B. A. (1995) 'Barriers to the diagnosis and treatment of depression in the community dwelling elderly', *Irish Journal of Psychological Medicine* 12: 22–3.

Lawlor, B., Radic, A., Bruce, I., Swanwick, G. R. J., O' Kelly, F., O' Doherty, M., Walsh, J. B. and Coakley, D. (1994) 'Prevalence of mental illness in an elderly community dwelling population using AGECAT', *Irish Journal of Psychological Medicine* 11 (4): 157–9.

Lee, E. (2001) 'The context of the post-abortion syndrome diagnosis', pp. 9–16 in *Psychological Sequelae of Abortion: The Myths and the Scientific Facts*. Bern: Symposium Inselspital.

Lee, E. (2003) *Abortion, Motherhood and Mental Health: Medicalizing Reproduction in the United States and Great Britain*. New York: Adeline de Gruyter.

Leff, J. (2001) 'Why is care in the community perceived a failure?', *British Journal of Psychiatry* 179: 381–3.

Lehmann, P. and Kempker, K. (1993) 'Unconventional approaches to psychiatry', *Clinical Psychology Forum* 51: 28–9.

Levy V., Robinson S. and Thomson A. M. (eds) (1993) *Midwives, Research and Childbirth*, vol. 3. London: Chapman & Hall.

Lonnqvist, J. K. (2000) 'Psychiatric aspects of suicidal behaviour: depression', pp. 107–20 in Hawton, K. and Van Heeringen, K. (eds), *The International Handbook of Suicide and Attempted Suicide*. Chichester: Wiley.

Lothian, K. and Philip, I. (2001) 'Maintaining the dignity and autonomy of older people in the healthcare setting', *British Medical Journal* 322: 668–70.

LRC (1993) *Consultation Paper on Sentencing*. Dublin: Law Reform Commission.

LRC (1996) *Report on Sentencing*. Dublin: Law Reform Commission.

Lynch, F., Mills, C., Daly, I. and Fitzpatrick, C. (2004) 'Challenging times: a study to detect Irish adolescents at risk of psychiatric disorders and suicidal ideation', *Journal of Adolescence* 27: 441–51.

Lynch, T. (2001) *Beyond Prozac: Healing Mental Suffering without Drugs*. Dublin: Marino.

MacDonald, A., Goddard, C. and Poynton, A. (1994). 'Impact of open access to specialist services: the case of community psychogeriatrics', *International Journal of Geriatric Psychiatry* 9: 709–14.

MacGabhann, L., Scheele, A., Dunne, T., Gallagher, P., MacNeela, P., Moore, G. and Philbin, M. (2004) *Mental Health Services and Addiction Services and the Management of Dual Diagnosis in Ireland*. Dublin: Stationery Office.

Madrid, H. M., Pombo, M. G. and Otero, A. G. (2001) 'Eating attitudes and body satisfaction in adolescence', *Psicothema* 13 (4): 539–45.

Magnusson, G. (2004) www. euro. who. int/mentalhealth/ChildAdolescent/.

Mangen, S. (1985) *Mental Health Care in the European Community*. London: Croom Helm.

Manning, N. (2001) 'Psychiatric diagnosis under conditions of uncertainty: personality disorder, sciences and professional legitimacy', pp. 76–94 in Busfield, J. (ed.), *Rethinking the Sociology of Mental Health*. Oxford: Blackwell.

Mansell, J and Ericsson, K. (eds) (1996) *Deinstitutionalization and Community Living: Intellectual Disability Services in Britain, Scandinavia and the USA*. London: Chapman Hall.

Marshall, M. (1996) 'Evaluation services for homeless people with mental disorders – theoretical and practical issues', pp 280–96 in Bhugra, D. (ed.), *Homelessness and Mental Health: Studies in Social and Community Psychiatry*. Cambridge: Cambridge University Press.

Marshall, M. (1998) 'Therapeutic buildings for people with dementia', pp. 11–14 in Judd S., Marshall, M. and Phippen, P. (eds), *Design for Dementia*. London: Journal of Dementia Care.

Martin, M., Carr, A., Carroll, L. and Byrne, S. (2005) 'Mental health service needs of children and adolescents in the south east of Ireland: a preliminary screening study', Dublin: 6th International Conference on Integrated Care, 14–15 Feb.

Mastronardi, M. (2003) 'Adolescence and media', *Journal of Language and Social Psychology* 22 (1): 83–93.

Mauthner, N., Killoran-Ross, M. and Brown, J. (1999) 'Mental health promotion theory and practice: insights from a literature review', *International Journal of Mental Health Promotion* 1 (1): 37–43.

McAuley, F. (1993) *Insanity, Psychiatry and Criminal Responsibility*. Dublin: Round Hall.

McCluskey, D. (1997) 'Conceptions of health and illness in Ireland', pp. 51–68 in Cleary A. and Treacy M. P. (eds), *The Sociology of Health and Illness in Ireland*. Dublin: UCD Press.

McEvoy, R. and Richardson, V. (2004) *Men's Health in Ireland*. The Men's Health Forum in Ireland, www.mhfi.org.

McGee, H., Garavan, R., de Barra, M., Byrne, J. and Conroy, R. (2002) *Sexual Abuse and Violence in Ireland (SAVI Report)*. Dublin: Liffey.

McGoran S. (1997) 'Lay perceptions of mental health: A collaborative project', pp. 255–60 in Trent D. A. and Reed C. A. (eds), *Promotion of Mental Health*, vol. 6. Aldershot: Ashgate.

McGowan, P. (2003) 'Future directions in peer counselling', Personal communication.

McGrath, E., Keita, G. P., Strickland, B. R. and Russo, N. F. (1990) *Women and Depression: Risk Factors and Treatment Issues*, Washington DC: American Psychological Association.

McKeon, P. (1999) *Public Attitudes to Depression: A National Survey*. Dublin: St Patrick's Hospital.

McKeon P. and Carrick, S. (1991) 'Public attitudes to depression: a national survey', *Irish Journal of Psychological Medicine* 8: 116–21.

McKeown, K. (1999) *Mentally Ill and Homeless in Ireland: Facing the Reality, Finding the Solutions*. Dublin: Disability Federation of Ireland.

McLoughlin, D. and McKeon, P. (1995) 'Employees attitude to depression – what they tell their boss', *Proceedings of World Federation of Mental Health, World Congress*, Dublin.

McNamee, P., Gregson, B., Buck, D., Bamford, C. H., Bond J. and Wright K. (1999) 'Cost of formal care for older people in England: the resource implications of the MRC cognitive function and ageing study', *Social Science and Medicine* 48: 331–41.

Mental Health Commission (2003) *Annual Report 2002*. Dublin: Stationery Office.

Mental Health Commission (2004a) *Annual Report 2003*. Dublin: Stationery Office.

Mental Health Commission (2004b) *Report of the Inspector of Mental Health Services 2003* Dublin: Stationery Office.

Mental Health Commission (2004c) *Mental Health Commission Strategic Plan 2004–5*. Dublin: Mental Health Commission.

Mental Health Ireland (2001) *Mental Health Matters: A Mental Health Resource Pack*. Dublin: Stationery Office.

Mentes, J. C. and Buckwalter, K. C. (1998) 'Dementia special care units: programming and staffing issues', *Journal of Gerontological Nursing*. Jan.: pp. 6–8.

Merwin, M. R. and Ochberg, F. M. (1983) 'The long voyage: policies for progress in mental health', *Health Affairs* 2 (4): 96–127.

Miller J. B. (1986) *Towards a New Psychology of Women*, 2nd edn. Boston: Beacon Press.

Miller, P. and Rose, N. (eds) (1986) *The Power of Psychiatry*. Cambridge: Polity.

Mind Out for Mental Health (2003) *Line Managers Resource a Practical Guide to Managing and Supporting Mental Health in the Workplace*. London: Department of Health.

Mitchell, J (1975) *Psychoanalysis and Feminism, Freud, Reich, Laing and Women*. New York: Vintage Books.

Mitchell, K. and Carr, A. (2002) 'Anorexia and bulimi', pp. 233–57 in Carr, A. (ed.), *Prevention: What Works with Children and Adolescents?* London: Routledge.

Muggivan, T. and Muggivan, J. J. (2004) *A Tragedy Waiting to Happen: The Chaotic Life of Brendan O'Donnell*. Dublin: Gill & Macmillan.

Murphy, G. E. (2000) 'Psychiatric aspects of suicidal behaviour: substance abuse', pp. 135–46 in Hawton, K. and Van Heeringen, K. (eds), *The International Handbook of Suicide and Attempted Suicide*. Chichester: Wiley.

Murphy-Lawless, J. (2002) 'Establishing the rationales for gender-specific strategies to improve women's health', unpublished paper.

National Assembly for Wales (2001), *The Welsh Office Key Health Statistics for Wales*. Government Statistical Service, Wales.

National Conjoint Child Health Committee (2000) *Getting Connected: Developing an Adolescent Friendly Health Service*. Dublin: Department of Health and Children.

National Crime Forum (1998) *Report*. Dublin: IPA.

NDA (2002) *Public Attitudes to Disability in the Republic of Ireland*. Dublin: NDA.

NDA (2003) *Review of Access to Mental Health Services for People with Intellectual Disabilities*. Dublin: NDA.

NESC (1987) *Community Care Services: An Overview*. Dublin: NESC.

NESF (2002) *Reintegration of Prisoners*, Forum Report no. 22. Dublin: NESF.

National Forensic Mental Health Service (2003) http://mentalhealthpolicy.ie/submissions/submission201.pdf

National Health and Medical Research Council (1999) *National Statement on Ethical Conduct in Research Involving Humans*, Canberra: NHMRC.

National Parasuicide Registry Ireland (2003) *Annual Report 2002*. Cork: National Suicide Research Foundation.

National Suicide Review Group (2001) *Suicide in Ireland: A National Study*. Navan: North Eastern Health Board.

Newman, B. M. and Newman, P. R. (2003) *Development Through Life: A Psychosocial Approach*, 8th edn. Australia: Thompson Wadsworth.

NHS Centre for Reviews and Dissemination (1997) 'Mental health promotion in high risk groups', *Effective Health Care Bulletin*: 3(3): 1–12.

Northern Area Health Board (2000) *Report of the Forum on Youth Homelessness*. Dublin: Northern Area Health Board.

NWCI (2003) *Women and Poverty*, Fact Sheet no. 2. Dublin. NWCI.

NWCI (2004) *Women and Paid Employment*, Fact Sheet, no. 1. Dublin. NWCI.

O'Brien, C. (2005) 'Rise in homelessness among mentally ill', *The Irish Times*, 1 Feb.

O'Brien, J., Carssow, K., Jones, M., Mercer, M., Reynolds, L. and Strzok, D. (2003) *Never Give Up: Assets Inc.'s Commitment to Community Life for People Seen as 'Difficult to Serve'*. Anchorage: Assets, Inc.

O'Connor, J. (1995) *The Workhouses of Ireland*. Dublin: Anvil.

ODEI the Equality Tribunal (2003) *Annual Report 2002*. Dublin: ODEI.

Office of Technology Assessment (OTA) (1990) *Confused Minds, Burdened Families: help for people with Alzheimer's and other dementias* (OTA Publication No BA-323). Washington DC: Congress of the United States.

Office of the Refugee Applications Commissioner (2004) *Monthly Statistics: August 2004 Issue*. Dublin: Office of the Refugee Applications Commissioner.

O'Gorman, A (2002) 'Overview of research on drug misuse among the homeless in Ireland', conference paper, *Homelessness and Problem Drug Use-Two Faces of Exclusion*. Dublin: Merchants Quay.

O'Hara, M. W., Wallace, R. B. and Kohort, F. J. (1985) 'Depression among the rural elderly: a study of prevalence and correlates', *Journal of Nervous and Mental Disorders* 173: 582–9.

O'Keane, V., Jeffers, A., Moloney, E. and Barry, S. (2003) *The Stark Facts: The Need for a National Mental Health Strategy*. Dublin: Irish Psychiatric Association.

O'Leary, J. (1997) *Beyond Help? Improving Service Provision for Street Homeless People with Mental Health and Alcohol or Drug Dependency Problems*. London: National Homeless Alliance.

Olfson, M., Mechanic, D., Hansell, S., Boyer, C. A. and Walkup, J. (1999) *Psychiatric Services* 50: 667–73.

Oliver, J., Huxley, P., Bridges, K. and Mohamad, H. (1996) *Quality of Life and Mental Health Services*. London: Routledge.

Oliver, M. and Barnes, C. (1998) *Disabled People and Social Policy: From Exclusion to Inclusion*. Harlow: Addison Wesley Longman.

O'Mahony, P. (1997) *Mountjoy Prisoners: A Sociological and Criminological Profile*. Dublin: Stationery Office.

O'Mahony, P. (ed) (2002a) *Criminal Justice in Ireland*. Dublin: IPA.

O'Mahony, P. (2002b) 'Introduction', pp. 3–10 in O'Mahony (ed.), *Criminal Justice in Ireland*. Dublin: IPA.

Onyett, S. (2003) *Teamworking in Mental Health*. Basingstoke: Palgrave Macmillan.

O'Shea, E. and O' Reilly, S. (1999) *An Action Plan on Dementia*, Report no. 54. Dublin: National Council on Ageing and Older People.

O'Sullivan, E. (1996) *Homelessness and Social Policy in the Republic of Ireland*. Occasional Paper no. 5, Department of Social Studies, TCD.

O'Sullivan, E. and Higgins, M. (2001) 'Women, the welfare state and homelessness in the Republic of Ireland', pp. 77–90 in Edgar, B. and Doherty, J. (eds), *Women and Homelessness in Europe: Pathways, Services and Experiences*. Bristol: Polity Press.

O'Sullivan, P. (2002) *Medico-Legal Reporting on Survivors of Torture in 2002*. Dublin: Centre for the Care of Survivors of Torture.

Paykel, E. S. (1991) 'Depression in women', *British Journal of Psychiatry* 10: 22–9.

Pear, R. (2003) 'Mental care poor for some children in state custody', *New York Times*, 1 Sept.

Peay, J. (2002) 'Mentally disordered offenders, mental health and crime', pp. 746–91 in Maguire, M., Morgan, R. and Reiner, R. (eds), *The Oxford Handbook of Criminology*, 3rd edn. Oxford: Oxford University Press.

Pigot, M. (1996) *Coping with Post-natal Depression; Light at the End of the Tunnel*. Dublin: Columba.

Pilgrim D. and A. Rogers (1999) *A Sociology of Mental Health and Illness*, 2nd edn. Buckingham: Open University Press.

Polivy, J., Herman, P., Mills, J. S. and Wheeler, H. B. (2003) 'Eating disorders in adolescence', pp. 523–49 in Adams, G. R. and Berzonsky, M. D. (eds), *Blackwell Handbook of Adolescence*. Oxford: Blackwell.

Powell, F. (1998) 'Mental health policy in the Republic of Ireland: backwards into the future', pp. 42–55 in J. Campbell and R. Manktelow (eds), *Mental Health Social Work in Ireland: Comparative Issues in Policy and Practice*. Aldershot: Ashgate.

Pratt, H. D., Phillips, E. L., Greydanus, D. E. and Patel, D. R. (2003) 'Eating disorders in the adolescent population: future directions', *Journal of Adolescent Research* 18 (3): 297–317.

Prior, P (1999) *Gender and Mental Health*. Basingstoke: Macmillan.

Psychological Society of Ireland (2003) *Submission to the Expert Group on Mental Health Services* Dublin: PSI.

Pugh, R. and Gould, N. (2000) 'Globalization, social work and social welfare', *European Journal of Social Work*, 3 (2): 123–38.

Putnam, R (2000) *Bowling Alone: The Collapse and Revival of American Community*. New York: Simon & Schuster.

Raeburn, R. and Rootman, B. (1998) *People-centred Health Promotion*. Chichester: Wiley.

Raftery, M. and O'Sullivan, E. (1999) *Suffer the Little Children: The Inside Story of Ireland's Industrial Schools*. Dublin: New Island.

Ramsay, R. and Gorst-Unsworth, C. (2003) 'Mental health problems in black refugees', pp. 201–21 in Ndegwa, D. and Olajide, Dele (eds), *Main Issues in Mental Health and Race*. Aldershot: Ashgate.

Rapp, C. and Wintersteen, R. (1989) 'The strengths model of case management', *Psychosocial Rehabilitation Journal* 13 (1): 23–32.

Regier, D. A., Narrow, W. E., Rae, D. S., Manderscheid, R. W., Locke, B. Z. and Goodwin, F. K. (1993) *The De Facto US Mental and Addictive Disorders, Service System. Epidemiological Catchment Area Prospective 1–Year Prevalence Rates of Disorders and Services*. Leicester: BPS Books.

Repper, J. and Cooney P. (1994) 'Meeting the needs of people with enduring mental health problems', in Thompson T. and Mathias P. (eds), *Lyttles Mental Health and Disorder*. London: Bailliere Tindall.

Rhodes, A and Goering, P (1998) 'Gender differences in the use of mental health services', pp. 19–33 in Lubotsky, B., Blanch, A. K. and Jennings, A. (eds), *Women's Mental Health Services: A Public Health Perspective*. California and London: Sage.

Richardson, B. and Orrell, M. (2002) 'Home assessments in old age psychiatry', *Advances in Psychiatric Treatment* 8: 59–65.

Ridley, J. and Jones, L. (2003) 'Direct what? The untapped potential of direct payments to mental health service users', *Disability and Society* 18 (5): 643–58.

Ritchie, K. and Kildea, D. (1995) 'Is senile dementia "age-related" or ageing-related: evidence from meta-analysis of dementia prevalence in the oldest old', *The Lancet* 346: 931– 4.

Robb, B. (1967) *Sans Everything: A Case to Answer.* London: Nelson.

Robins, J (1986) *Fools and Mad: A History of the Insane in Ireland.* Dublin: IPA.

Rogers, A. and Pilgrim, D. (2001) *Mental Health Policy in Britain*, 2nd edn. Houndmills: Palgrave.

Romito, P and Guerin, D (2000) 'Asking patients about violence, a survey of 510 women attending social and health services in Trieste, Italy' *Social Science and Medicine* 54 (12): 1813–24.

Rosenthal, R. (1994) *Homelessness in Paradise: A Map of the Terrain*, Philadelphia: Temple University Press.

Rowe, J. W. and Kahn, R. L. (1998) *Successful Ageing.* New York: Pantheon.

Royal College of Obstetrics and Gynaecology (2004) *National Evidence-Based Clinical Guidelines: The Care of Women Requesting Induced Abortion* (www. rcog. org. uk).

Royal College of Psychiatrists (2003) *Asylum-seekers, Refugees and Mental Health in the UK: Position Statement of the Transcultural Special Interest Group.* London: Royal College of Psychiatrists.

Ruddle, H. (1998) 'The review findings' in *Review of the Implementation of Recommendations of The Years Ahead: A Policy for The Elderly and Implications for Future Policy on Older People on Ireland*, Report no. 49. Dublin: National Council on Ageing and Older People.

Ruddle, H., Donoghue, F. and Mulvihill, R. (1997) *The Years Ahead Report: A Review of the Implementation of its Recommendations*, Report no. 48. Dublin: National Council on Ageing and Older People.

Rue, V (1995) 'Post-abortion syndrome: a variant of post-traumatic stress disorder', pp. 15–28 in Doherty, P. (ed.), *Post-abortion Syndrome: Its Wider Ramifications.* Dublin. Four Courts.

Rusiecki, W. and Alfinito, M. (1997) 'Cross cultural integration: using case management to bridge the gap for individuals with dual diagnosis', pp. 1–5 in Fletcher, R. J. (ed.), *The NADD Newsletter Book.* New York: National Association for the Dually Diagnosed.

Rutter, D. L., Quine, L. and Chesham, D. J. (1993) *Social Psychological Approaches to Health and Safety.* New York: Harvester Wheatsheaf.

Rutter, M. and Smith, D. (1995) *Psychosocial Disorders in Young People: Time Trends and Their Causes.* Chichester: Wiley.

Rutz, W. (2001) 'Mental health in Europe: problems, advances and challenges'. *Acta Psychiatrica Scandinavica* 104 (suppl. 410): 15–20.

Sainsbury Centre for Mental Health (2003a) *The Economic and Social Costs of Mental Illness.* London: Sainsbury Centre for Mental Health.

Sainsbury Centre for Mental Health (2003b) *Mental Health Service User Movement in England*, London: Sainsbury Centre for Mental Health.

Santrock, J. W. (2002) *Life-Span Development*, 8th issue. Boston: McGraw Hill.

Saris, A. J. (1997) 'The asylum in Ireland: a brief institutional history and some local effects', pp. 208–23 in Cleary, A. and Treacy, M. P. (eds), *The Sociology of Health and Illness in Ireland.* Dublin: UCD Press.

Sartorius, N. (1998) 'Universal strategies for the prevention of mental illness and the promotion of mental health', pp. 61–7 in Jenkins, R. and Ustun, T. B. (eds), *Preventing Mental illness: Mental Health Promotion in Primary Care.* Chichester: Wiley.

Scheff, T. (1981) 'The role of the mentally ill and the dynamics of mental disorder: a research framework', pp. 54–62 in Grusky O. and Pollner, M. (eds), *The Sociology of Mental Illness: Basic Studies.* Orlando: Holt, Rinehart & Winston.

Scottish Executive (2001) *National Programme for Improving Mental Health and Well-being.* (Edinburgh: Scottish Executive).

Scottish Executive (2003) *National Programme for Improving Mental Health and Well-being Action Plan 12003–2006* (Edinburgh: Scottish Executive).

Scull, A. (1977) *Decarceration: Community Treatment and the Deviant: A Radical View.* Cambridge: Polity.

Secker, J. (1998) 'Current conceptualisations of mental health and mental health promotion', *Health Education Research* 13 (1): 57–66.

Sedgwick, P. (1982) *Psycho Politics.* London: Pluto.

Seedhouse, D. (1986) *Health: The Foundations for Achievement.* Chichester: Wiley.

Shatkin, J. and Belfer, M. (2004) 'The global absence of child and adolescent mental health policy', *Children and Adolescent Mental Health* 9 (3): 104–10.

Silverstone, B. (2000) 'The old and the new in aging: implications for social work practice', *Journal of Gerontological Social Work* 33 (4): 33–50.

Slate, R. (2003) 'From the jailhouse to Capitol Hill: impacting mental health court legislation and defining what constitutes a mental health court', *Crime and Delinquency* 49 (1): 6–29

Sluzki, C. E. (1979) 'Migration and family conflict', *Family Process* 18 (4): 379–90.

Smaje, C. (1996) 'The ethnic patterning of health: new directions for theory and research', *Sociology of Health and Illness* 18 (2): 139–71.

Smith, J. (1981) 'The idea of health: a philosophical inquiry', *Advances in Nursing Science* 3 (3): 43–50.

Smith, C., O'Neill, H., Tobin, J. and Walshe, D. (1996) 'Mental disorders detected in an Irish prison sample', *Criminal Behaviour and Mental Health* 6: 177–83.

Smith, J. (1999) 'Gender and homelessness', pp. 108–32 in Hutson, S. and Clapham D. (eds), *Homelessness: Public Policies and Private Troubles.* London, New York: Cassell.

Smith, M., McGee, H, Shannon, W. and Holohan, T. (2001) *One Hundred Homeless Women: Health Status and Health Service Use of Homeless Women and Their Children in Dublin.* Dublin: Royal College of Surgeons in Ireland and the Eastern Region Health Authority.

Smith, R. (1981) *Trial by Medicine: Insanity and Responsibility in Victorian Trials.* Edinburgh: Edinburgh University Press.

Smyth, C., MacLachlan, M. and Clare, A. (2003) *Cultivating Suicide: Destruction of Self in a Changing Ireland.* Dublin: Liffey.

Snow, David A. and Anderson, L. (1993): *Down on Their Luck: A Study of Homeless Street People.* Berkeley, CA: University of California Press.

Social Exclusion Unit (2004) *Mental Health and Social Exclusion, Social Exclusion Unit Report.* London: Office of the Deputy Prime Minister.

Solomon, B. (2001) 'Mental health services to ethnic minorities: a global perspective', pp. 189–212 in Dominelli, L., Lorenz, W. and Soydan, H. (eds), *Beyond Racial Divides: Ethnicities in Social Work Practice.* Aldershot: Ashgate.

South Western Area Health Board (2001) *A Review of the Needs and Services for Children and Young People with Asperger's in the Area Health Boards of the Eastern Region.* Naas: SWAHB.

STAKES (1998) *Promotion of Mental Health on the European Agenda: Consultative Meeting.* Helsinki: National Research and Development Centre for Welfare and Health.

STAKES (1999a) 'Introduction to mental health issues in the EU' www. stakes. fi/mentalhealth/introduction. htm.

STAKES (1999b) Mental health policies in the member states', www. stakes/fi/mentalhealth/ Questionnare. htm.

STAKES (2005) *Implementing Mental Health Promotion Action.* www.preventioncentre.net/ imhpa

Stokes, G. and Goudie, F. (1990) *Working with Dementia.* Bicester: Winslow.

Stone, T. H. (1997) 'Therapeutic implications of incarceration for persons with severe mental disorders: searching for rational health policy', *American Journal of Criminal Law* 24: 283–358.

Stoppard, J. M. (2000) *Understanding Depression: Feminist Social Constructionist Approaches.* London and New York: Routledge.

Stotland, Nada (2004) Nada Stotland, Professor of Psychiatry and Professor of Obstetrics and Gynaecology at Rush Medical College, testimony to US House of Representatives.

Strathdee, G. and Jenkins, R. (1996) 'Purchasing mental health care for primary care', pp. 71–84 in Thornicroft, G. and Strathdee, G. (eds), *Commissioning Mental Health Services,* London: HMSO.

Stubbs, P. (1993) '"Ethnically sensitive" or "anti-racist"? Models for health research and service delivery', pp. 34–47 in Ahmad, W. I. U. (ed.), *'Race' and Health in Contemporary Britain.* Buckingham: Open University Press.

Study Group on the Development of the Psychiatric Services (1984) *The Psychiatric Services: Planning for the Future.* Dublin: Stationery Office.

Sullivan, G., Burnam, A. and Koegel, P. (2000) 'Pathways to homelessness among the mentally ill', *Social Psychiatry and Psychiatric Epidemiology* 35: 444–50.

Summerfield, D. (1996) *The Impact of War and Atrocity on Civilian Populations: Basic Principles for NGO Interventions and a Critique of Psychosocial Trauma Projects.* Relief and Rehabilitation Network: Network Paper 14. London: Overseas Development Institute.

Swanwick, G. R. J. and Lawlor, B. (1998) 'Services for dementia suffers and their carers: implications for future development', pp. 199–220, in Leahy, A. L. and Wiley, M. (eds), *The Irish Health System in the 21st Century.* Dublin: Oak Tree.

Swanwick, G. R. J., Coen, R. F. and O'Mahoney, D. (1996) 'A memory clinic for the assessment of mild dementia', *Irish Medical Journal* 89: 104–5.

Szasz, T. (1961) *The Myth of Mental Illness.* New York: Harper & Row.

Szasz T. (1981) 'The myth of mental illness', pp. 45–54 in Grusky O. and Pollner M. (eds), *The Sociology of Mental Illness: Basic Studies.* Orlando: Holt, Rinehart & Winston.

Szasz, T. S. (1987) 'The psychiatric will: a new mechanism for the protection of persons against 'psychosis' and psychiatry', *American Psychologist* 37 (7): 762–9.

Tester, S. (1996) *Community Care for Older People: A Comparative Perspective.* London: Macmillan.

Tew, J. (2002) 'Going social: championing a holistic model of mental distress within professional education', *Social Work Education* 1 (2): 143–56.

Thai, H. C. (2002) 'Clashing dreams: highly educated overseas and low wage US husbands', pp. 230–53 in Ehrenreich, B. and Hochschild, A. R. (eds), *Global Woman: Nannies, Maids and Sex Workers in the New Economy.* London: Granta.

Tilford, S., Delaney, F., Vogels, M. and Meyrick, J. (eds) (1997) *Effectiveness of Mental Health Promotion Interventions: A Review.* London: HEA.

Timms, P. (1993) 'Mental health and homelessness', pp. 94–116 in Fisher, K and Collins, J. (eds), *Homelessness, Health Care and Welfare Provision.* London: Routledge.

Timms, P. and Fry, A. H. (1989) 'Homelessness and mental illness', *Health Trends* 21: 70–1.

Townsend, P. (1962) *The Last Refuge: A Survey of Residential Institutions and Homes for the Aged in England and Wales.* London: Routledge & Kegan Paul.

Townsend, P. (1986) 'Ageism and social policy', pp. 15–45, in Phillipson, C. and Walker, A. (eds), *Ageing and Social Policy: A Critical Assessment.* Aldershot: Gower.

Trent, D. (1992) 'Breaking the single continuum', pp. 117–26 in Trent, D. R. (ed.), *Promotion of Mental Health*, vol. 1. Aldershot: Avebury..

Trent, D. (1994) 'Fighting the four horsemen', pp. 377–84 in Trent, D. R. and Reed, C. (eds), *Promotion of Mental Health*, vol. 3. Aldershot: Avebury.

Tudor, K. (1996) *Mental Health Promotion Paradigms and Practice.* London: Routledge.

Turner, C. B. and Kramer, B. M. (1995) 'Connections between racism and mental health', pp. 3–26 in Willie, C. V., Ricker, P. P., Kramer, B. M. and Brown, B. S. (eds), *Mental Health, Racism and Sexism.* London: Taylor & Francis.

UK Department of Health (2002) Women's Mental Health: Into the Mainstream, Strategic Development of Mental Health Care for Women. London: Department of Health Publications.

UK Department of Health (2003) Health and personal social services statistics section: Table B16 hospital inpatient activity: average daily number of available beds by sector, NHS trusts [online], Available: http://www. doh. gov. uk/hpsss/index. htm.

UN Committee on the Rights of the Child (1998) 453rd meeting CRC/C/15 Add. 85.

UN High Commissioner for Human Rights (2001) To the Economic and Social Council. UN Doc. no. E/2001//64.

United Nations (1989) *Convention on the Rights of the Child.* New York: UN.

United Nations (1990) *Standard Minimum Rules for Non-custodial Measures (The Tokyo Rules).* Adopted by General Assembly resolution 45/110 of Dec. 1990: New York: United Kingdom.

United Nations (1994) *Standard Rules for the Equalisation of Opportunities for Persons with Disabilities.* New York: UN.

United Nations (2002) *Report of the Committee on Economic, Social and Cultural Rights.* New York: UN.

United Nations Committee on the Rights of the Child (1998) 453rd Meeting 23 Jan. CRC/C/15Add. 85.

United States General Accounting Office (2002) *Welfare Reform – Outcomes for TANF Recipients with Impairments,* GAO Report 02–884 and GAO, WASHINGTON DC.

US Department of Health and Human Services (1999) *Mental Health: A Report of the Surgeon General: Executive Summary.* Rockville MD: US Department of Health and Human Services, Substance Abuse and Mental Health Services Administration, Centre for Mental Health Services, National Institutes of Health, National Institute of Mental Health.

Ussher, J. M. (1992) 'Science sexing psychology', pp. 39–67 in Ussher, J. M. and Nicholson, P. (eds), *Gender Issues in Clinical Psychology.* London: Routledge.

Ussher, J. M. (2000) 'Women and mental illness', pp. 77–90 in Sherr, L. and St Lawrence, J. (eds), *Women, Health and the Mind*. Chichester: Wiley.

Vaillant, G. E. (2003) 'Mental health', *American Journal of Psychiatry* 160 (8): 1373–84.

Vaillant, G. E. and Blumenthal, S. J. (1990) 'Introduction: suicide over the life cycle: risk factors and life-span development', pp. 1–14 in Blumenthal S. J. and Kupfer D. J. (eds), *Suicide Over the Life Cycle: Risk Factors, Assessment and Treatment of Suicidal Patients*. Washington: American Psychiatric Press.

Vaillant, G. E. and Mukamal, K. (2001) 'Successful aging', *American Journal of Psychiatry* 156 (6): 839–47.

Videbeck, S. L. (2001) *Psychiatric Mental Health Nursing*. Philadelphia: Lippincott Williams & Wilkins.

Vincent, M. A. and McCabe, M. P. (1999) 'Gender differences among adolescents in family and peer influences on body dissatisfaction, weight loss and binge eating behaviours', *Adolescence* 30: 205–21.

Vitiello, B. and Behar, D. (1992) 'Mental retardation and psychiatric illness', *Hospital and Community Psychiatry* 43: 494–9.

Von Abendorff, R., Challis, D. and Netten, A. (1994) 'Staff activity patterns in a community mental health team for older people', *International Journal of Geriatric Psychiatry* 9: 897–906.

Vostanis, P., Grattan, E. and Cumella, S. (1998) 'Mental health problems of homeless children and families: longitudinal study', *British Medical Journal* 21 316 (7135): 899–902.

Waaddegaard, M. and Peterson, T. (2002) 'Dieting and desire for weight loss among adolescents in Denmark: a questionnaire survey', *European Eating Disorders Review* 10 (5): 329–46.

Waddington, L. and Hendriks, A. (2002) 'The expanding concept of employment discrimination in Europe: from direct and indirect discrimination to reasonable accommodation', *International Journal of Comparative Labour Law and Industrial Relations*, 18 (3): 403–27.

Wahl, O. F. (2003) 'News media portrayal of mental illness. implications for public policy', *American Behavioral Scientist* 46 (12): 1594–1600.

Walker, A. (1986) 'The politics of ageing' pp 30–45, in Phillipson, C., Bernard, M. and Strang, P. (eds), *Dependency and Interdependency in Old Age-Theoretical Perspectives and Policy Alternatives*. London: Croom Helm.

Walker, A. (1993) 'Community care policy: from consensus to conflict', pp. 204–26 in Bornat, J. et al. (eds), *Community Care: A Reader*. Basingstoke: Macmillan.

Walker, N. (1968) *Crime and Insanity in England* 1: *The Historical Perspective*. Edinburgh: Edinburgh University Press.

Walker, A. and Maltby. T. (1997) *Ageing Europe*. Buckingham: Open University Press.

Walsh, D. (1987) 'Recent trends in mental health care in Ireland', *International Journal of Mental Health* 16 (1–2): 108–17.

Walsh, D. (2004) *Report of the Inspector of Mental Hospitals for the Year Ending 31st December 2003*, Dublin: Stationery Office.

Warner, M., Furnish, S., Lawlor, B., Longley, M., Sime, C. and Kelleher, M. (1998) *European Transnational Alzheimer's Study (ETAS). European Analysis of Public Health Policy Developments for Alzheimer's Disease and Associated Disorders of Older People and their Carers*. Brussels: European Commission, Directorate General V, Directorate of Public Health and Safety at Work.

Warren, J. W., Sobal, J., Tenney, J. H., Hoopes, J. M., Damron, D., Levenson, S., DeForge, B. R. and Muncie, H. L. (1986) 'Informed consent by proxy: an issue in research with elderly patients', *New England Journal of Medicine* 315: 1124–8.

Watters, C. (1996) 'Representations of Asians' mental health in British psychiatry', pp. 88–105 in Samson, C. and South, N. (eds), *The Social Construction of Social Policy: Methodologies, Racism, Citizenship and the Environment.* Basingstoke: Macmillan.

Watters, C. (1998) 'The mental health needs of refugees and asylum seekers: key issues in research and service development', pp. 282–97 in Nicholson, F. and Twomey, P. (eds), *Current Issues of UK Asylum Law and Policy.* Aldershot: Ashgate.

Watts, C. and Zimmerman, C. (2002) 'Violence against women: global scale and magnitude', *The Lancet.* 359, 6 Apr.: 1232–7.

Webb, M., McClelland, R. and Mock, G. (2002) 'Psychiatric services in Ireland: North and South'. *Irish Journal of Psychological Medicine* 19 (1): 21–6.

Weissmann, M. M., Bland, R., Joyce, P. R., Newman, S., Wells, J. E. and Wittchen, H. (1993) 'Sex differences in rates of depression: cross national perspectives', *Journal of Affective Disorders* 29: 77–84.

Weller, M. P. (1986) 'Medical concepts in psychopathy and violence', *Medicine, Science and the Law* 26 (2): 131–43.

Wells J. S. G. (2004) 'Community mental health policy in the 1990s: a case study in corporate and 'street level' implementation'. Unpublished PhD thesis, University of London.

Wertheim, E. H., Koerner, J. and Paxton, S. J. (2001) 'Longitudinal predictors of restrictive eating and bulimic tendencies in three different age groups of adolescent girls', *Adolescence* 29 (2): 69–81.

WHO (1977) *Child Mental Health and Psychosocial Development: Report of a WHO Expert Committee.* Geneva: WHO.

WHO (1978) *Primary Health Care, Alma Ata Conference.* Geneva: WHO.

WHO (1984) *Health Promotion: A WHO Discussion Document on the Concepts and Principles.* Geneva: WHO.

WHO (1991) *Health for All Targets: The Health Policy for Europe.* Copenhagen: WHO.

WHO (1986a) *Ottawa Charter for Health Promotion.* Geneva: WHO.

WHO (1996b) *Mental Health Care Law: Ten Basic Principles.* Geneva: WHO

WHO (1998) *Health Promotion Evaluation: Recommendations to Policy Makers.* Geneva: WHO.

WHO (1999) *Health for All in the 21st Century.* Geneva: WHO.

WHO (2001a) *The World Health Report 2001 – Mental Health: New Understanding, New Hope.* Geneva: WHO.

WHO (2001b) *Mental Health: A Call for Action by World Health Ministers.* Geneva: WHO.

WHO (2001c) *Mental Health Policy Project.* Geneva: WHO.

WHO (2002a) *Prevention and Promotion in Mental Health Mental Health: Evidence and Research.* Geneva: WHO.

WHO (2002b) *World Health Report 2002.* Geneva: WHO

WHO (2002c) *World Health Report on Violence and Health.* Geneva: WHO

WHO (2003) *Caring for Children and Adolescents with Mental Health Disorders: Setting WHO Directions.* Geneva: WHO.

WHO (2004a) *Pre-Conference on Mental Health of Children and Adolescents.* Geneva: WHO.

WHO (2004b) www.who.int/mental_health/prevention/childado/en/

WHO (2005a) *Child and Adolescent Mental Health Policies and Plans.* Geneva: WHO.

WHO (2005b) *Mental Health Declaration for Europe: Facing the Challenges, Building Solutions.* Helsinki: WHO Ministerial Conference, 12–15 January 2005, EUR/04/5047810/6. Geneval: WHO.

WHO with Victoria Health Promotion Foundation and University of Melbourne (2004) *Promoting Mental Health Concepts: Emerging Evidence Practice.* Geneva: WHO.

Williams, C. (2003) *From Social Care To Social Inclusion.* York: Northern Centre for Mental Health.

Williams, J and Gorby, S. (2002) *Counted in 2002: The Report of the Assessment of Homelessness in Dublin.* Dublin: ESRI and the Homeless Agency.

Williams, J. and O'Connor, M. (1999) *Counted In: The Report of the 1999 Assessment of Homelessness in Dublin, Kildare and Wicklow.* Dublin: Homeless Initiative.

Williams, R. and Avebury, K. A. (1995) *A Place in Mind: Commissioning and Providing Mental Health Services for People who are Homeless.* London: HMSO.

Women's Health Council (2002) *Promoting Women's Health: A Population Investment for Ireland's Future.* Dublin: Women's Health Council.

Women's Health Council (2004) *Women, Disadvantage and Health: A position paper of the Women's Health Council.* Dublin: Women's Health Council.

Woodcock, J. (1995) 'Healing rituals with families in exile', *Journal of Family Therapy* 17: 397–409.

Zaider, T. I., Johnson, J. G. and Cockell, S. J. (2002) 'Psychiatric disorders associated with the onset and persistence of bulimia nervosa and binge eating disorder during adolescence', *Journal of Youth and Adolescence* 31 (5): 319–29.

Ziglio, E., Hagard, S. and J. Griffiths (2000) 'Health promotion development in Europe: achievements and challenges', *Health Promotion International* 15: 143–54.

Index